10 Tips

on
Foot Care
for
People
with
Diabetes

2nd Edition

Jessie H. Ahroni, PhD, ARNP, CDE, BC-ADM
Neil M. Scheffler, DPM, FACFAS, FAPWCA

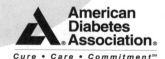

American Diabetes Association.
Cure • Care • Commitment℠

Director, Book Publishing, John Fedor; *Managing Editor,* Abe Ogden; *Book Acquisitions,* Robert Anthony; *Editor,* Rebecca Lanning; *Production Manager,* Melissa Sprott; *Cover Design,* Bremmer & Goris; *Printer,* Worzalla Publishing.

Printed in the United States of America
1 3 5 7 9 10 8 6 4 2

⊚ The paper in this publication meets the requirements of the ANSI Standard Z39.48-1992 (permanence of paper).

ADA titles may be purchased for business or promotional use or for special sales. To purchase this book in large quantities, or for custom editions of this book with your logo, contact Lee Romano Sequeira, Special Sales & Promotions, at the address below, or at LRomano@ diabetes.org or 703-299-2046.

American Diabetes Association
1701 North Beauregard Street
Alexandria, Virginia 22311

Library of Congress Cataloging-in-Publication Data

Ahroni, Jessie H., 1948–
    101 tips on foot care for people with diabetes / Jessie H. Ahroni and Neil M. Scheffler.—2nd ed.
    p. cm.
    Rev. ed. of: 101 foot care tips for people with diabetes. c2000.
    Includes bibliographical references and index.
    ISBN 1-58040-249-6 (alk. paper)
    1. Foot—Diseases—Popular works. 2. Diabetes—Complications. 3. Self-care, Health. I. Title: One hundred and one tips on foot care for people with diabetes. II. Scheffler, Neil M. III. Ahroni, Jessie H., 1948– . 101 foot care tips for people with diabetes. IV. Title.
    RC951.A38 2006
    617.5'85—dc22
                                                    2005035460

Contents

Preface

One of the greatest fears for people with diabetes is that they will lose a foot or a leg to amputation. This is a valid concern; each year, more than 80,000 of these amputations are performed. With proper care, however, your feet can and should last a lifetime. So what, exactly, does this care consist of? What can you do at home, and when do you need a doctor's help? How do you decide what care is right for you? How can you and your medical team work together to keep your feet intact? This book aims to help you answer these and many other questions.

In my work as a podiatrist for over three decades, I have treated the feet of thousands of people. One of the many lessons I have learned from my patients is that the ones who do the best are the ones who are attentive to their feet, who ask questions, who listen and learn and follow up. I hope this book will help you do all these things—and will help keep you healthy and walking comfortably.

Neil M. Scheffler, DPM, FACFAS, FAPWCA
Baltimore, Maryland

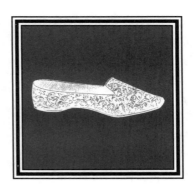

Chapter 1
General Tips

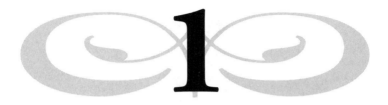

Why is it important for me to take special care of my feet?

If you want to be active and independent all of your life—whether or not you have diabetes—you need to have healthy feet. Most people take their feet for granted, but people with diabetes really cannot do that. You are challenged by two complications of diabetes that can affect the nerves and blood vessels of the feet—diabetic nerve damage and poor circulation. These complications make it easier for you to get a foot ulcer that may not heal. Non-healing ulcers often lead to amputation, which severely limits what you can do for yourself.

The good news is that by taking good care of your feet, you can often prevent diabetic foot complications. If you take care of your feet every day and get good medical care as soon as you even suspect that you might need it, you're much more likely to avoid getting the infections that make amputation necessary. In fact, at least 50% of amputations in people with diabetes could be prevented in this way. You can protect your feet.

What foot problems do people with diabetes experience?

People with diabetes have the same foot problems that people without diabetes experience—corns, calluses, bunions, ingrown toenails, arthritis, and broken bones. However, these ordinary foot problems can be more serious in people with diabetes if they also have diabetic nerve disease or poor circulation.

People with diabetic nerve damage cannot feel their feet, so they may not notice an injury, sores, or even high-pressure areas on their feet. They may continue to walk on an injury or high-pressure spot that would cause pain in a person without nerve damage. This continued walking might cause a wound or ulcer. Once the skin is broken, the ulcer can become infected. The blood supply carries oxygen, white blood cells that attack bacteria, and healing nutrients to wounds. It also carries any antibiotics that you take. But if you don't have enough blood supply to the foot, an ulcer can be difficult or impossible to heal. If not treated, some of these foot infections lead to amputation.

Am I more likely to get an infection just because I have diabetes?

Yes. People with diabetes who have high blood glucose levels most of the time are more likely to develop infections than people with normal blood glucose levels. High blood glucose can interfere with your body's natural defense systems so that infections are harder to heal, too.

Healthy skin is your main defense against infection, and diabetes can make your skin dry and more susceptible to cracking. Once the skin is broken, germs can enter. Fungal diseases that appear in folds of skin and on your feet need glucose and moisture to grow, and they like high blood glucose levels. The damage they do to your skin can allow an infection to begin.

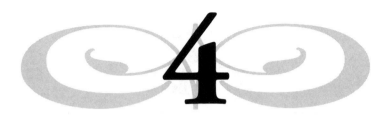

How common are diabetic foot problems?

The short answer is, way too common. About half of the people who have had diabetes for 10 years have some degree of nerve damage. The older you are and the longer you have had diabetes, the more likely you are to have nerve damage—but not everybody gets it. Recent studies show that people who keep their blood glucose levels close to normal are less likely to develop nerve damage or poor blood circulation.

It is estimated that 15–25% of people with diabetes will have a foot ulcer at least once. About 70% of these ulcers will heal with good basic foot care. Up to 10% of people with diabetes will have an amputation at some time in their lives. Toe and partial foot amputations are the most common, followed by below-the-knee amputations. Amputation rates are greater with increasing age, in males compared with females, and among African Americans and Hispanic Americans. Experts believe that at least half of these amputations could be prevented by near-normal blood glucose levels, better preventive foot care, and better care of foot ulcers.

Who is at greatest risk for diabetic foot problems?

The people most at risk have diabetic nerve damage. If poor circulation is also present, the danger increases. Other risk factors include limited joint mobility, foot deformity or thick nails, a history of having a foot ulcer or amputation, or having other complications of diabetes, such as eye disease (retinopathy) or kidney disease (nephropathy). Once you have had a foot ulcer or amputation, you are likely to get another one. This is because you have serious damage to the nerves and blood vessels of your feet, not because you do not take care of your feet. Most people with diabetes who have had foot problems take better than average care of their feet, but good foot care alone may not be enough to prevent foot problems once they are already established.

Newly diagnosed young people with type 1 diabetes who do not have other complications of diabetes or other foot problems have little risk. The American Diabetes Association recommends that annual foot risk screening begin 5 years after the diagnosis of diabetes, but it is never too early to develop good foot care habits.

Older people who are recently diagnosed with type 2 diabetes may actually have had diabetes for years before finding out about it and may already have complications. If you have type 2 diabetes, start good foot care right away.

What can I do to prevent diabetic foot problems?

- Look at and touch your feet every day: tops, bottoms, backs, sides, and between the toes. Get prompt medical attention for any problems.
- Keep your feet clean and dry.
- Cut or file toenails with the shape of the toe, smoothing all sharp edges.
- Moisturize dry skin with a good lotion.
- Avoid injury to your feet. Have corns, calluses, or ingrown toenails treated by a podiatrist.
- Wear well-fitting socks, without a thick toe seam, made of a material that wicks moisture away from the skin, such as acrylic or CoolMax.
- Wear well-fitting soft leather or fabric shoes, such as running shoes. Wear house shoes at home. Never go barefoot.
- Check shoes daily for cracks, pebbles, or other things that might damage your feet.
- Try to keep your blood glucose levels near normal.
- Have surgery to fix deformities such as bunions and hammertoes.

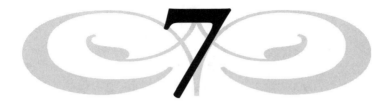

Does my weight affect my feet?

Absolutely. This is just common sense, and not just for people with diabetes. The more we weigh, the more stress is transmitted through our knees, ankles, and feet. Many people with foot pain can get relief just by losing weight. Heel pain is one example of a pain that is often weight related. Arthritis pain in the knees and feet is frequently worse in people who are overweight.

People who are obese have a different gait from those who are not. Their feet are placed wider than normal because their thighs hold the legs outward. This places the body weight more toward the inner part of the foot, changing the mechanics of walking completely. There is increased stress on the tendons, ligaments, and joints of the feet.

If you have diabetic neuropathy, your weight is even more important. The stress of additional pounds on numb feet increases the likelihood of your developing ulcers and Charcot deformities.

If you become pregnant, your feet may change shape and size during the pregnancy and for about 6 months after the baby is born. Sometimes they remain permanently larger. Be aware of this and try to wear comfortable, supportive shoes, such as running shoes. High heels are not really a good idea for anyone, but especially not for a pregnant woman.

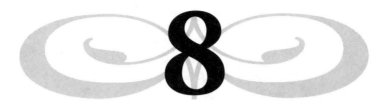

What do blood glucose levels have to do with feet?

If you can keep your blood glucose levels close to normal, you decrease your chances of getting diabetic complications. If you already have complications, you may keep them from getting worse or slow down their progression. With near-normal blood glucose levels, you are less likely to develop nerve damage or poor circulation, and you'll heal faster.

Results from the two largest studies of blood glucose management, the Diabetes Control and Complications Trial (DCCT) and the United Kingdom Prospective Diabetes Study (UKPDS), support this. The DCCT studied 1,400 people with type 1 diabetes. Half of the people received "conventional" care (1–2 insulin injections a day), and the other half received "intensive" care (as many injections as needed to keep blood glucose levels close to the normal range). Patients with near-normal blood glucose levels had a 40–70% reduction in the complications of diabetes. This improvement occurred regardless of the patients' age, sex, or length of time they'd had diabetes.

The UKPDS studied the effects of near-normal blood glucose levels in 5,200 people with type 2 diabetes by placing them in conventional (diet and exercise) or intensive (oral medications or insulin) care groups. The results were dramatic and showed the same strong benefits of near-normal blood glucose levels in preventing or slowing down diabetic complications.

I've heard about the "team approach" to treating diabetes. What kind of team do I need for my foot health?

The most important member of the team is YOU. You need to practice good foot hygiene, wear your prescribed shoes and inserts, and in general take charge of your own foot health. The other members of your foot care team will probably include a primary health care provider and a podiatrist (foot specialist). They may suggest other team members:

- Vascular surgeons can help restore circulation to the feet. They specialize in surgery on the blood vessels.
- A neurologist may join the team if you have neuropathy.
- A physiatrist (specialist in rehabilitation medicine) and a physical or occupational therapist may be consulted if you need rehabilitation.
- A pedorthist is a professional shoe fitter who makes and fits shoes and insoles for people with foot problems. Pedorthists can be helpful if you have lost feeling in your feet. When you visit a pedorthist make sure you have your doctor's prescription or recommendation with you.
- A certified diabetes educator (CDE) can help teach you how to care for your feet.
- An endocrinologist can help with your diabetes management.
- Your family members who help you care for your feet at home can also be part of the team.

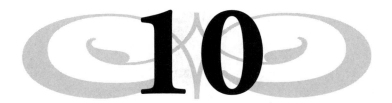

How do I know whether to see a podiatrist or an orthopedic surgeon?

Ask your health care provider. You can see a podiatrist for routine foot care if you cannot see well or reach your feet. Podiatrists are doctors of podiatric medicine (DPM) and, in most states, diagnose and treat conditions of the feet and ankles. They perform routine foot care, such as toenail trimming, callus removal, and treatment for ingrown toenails, and they perform foot surgery on bones and soft tissue, such as bunion or hammertoe surgery. They can study how your feet and legs work when you move and walk (biomechanics). They can pinpoint bones that are out of place and that put unusual pressure on the skin of your feet. They can design insoles or braces to help your feet work normally and order special footwear if you need it. Podiatrists are trained in the treatment of the diabetic foot, including the treatment of wounds and infections.

Orthopedic surgeons are medical doctors (MD) who perform surgery on the bones. Some may concentrate on foot and ankle problems. Orthopedic surgeons do not usually provide routine services such as toenail trimming and removing ingrown toenails. They may perform foot surgery. They too can order arch supports, braces, and special footwear if you need it.

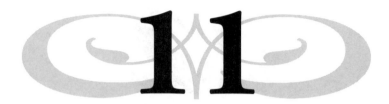

How often should I have a doctor take care of my feet?

Have a complete foot examination at least once a year. Your health care provider or podiatrist will look for any changes in shape (deformity) that alter the way you walk and bear weight on the foot. He or she will also check for loss of feeling by pressing a thin plastic wire called a monofilament against the soles of your feet or by holding a vibrating tuning fork against the base of your big toe. The provider will check your circulation and examine your skin, especially between your toes and under the metatarsal heads (the bones in the ball of your foot).

If you can't examine your own feet or if you have foot problems or nerve damage, have your feet checked more often, probably at every visit to your health care provider.

The following are warning signs to have your feet checked even sooner:

- redness, swelling, or increased warmth
- a change in the size or shape of the foot or ankle
- pain in the legs at rest or while walking
- open sores with or without drainage, no matter how small
- nonhealing wounds
- ingrown toenails
- corns or calluses with skin discoloration
- unexplained high blood glucose levels

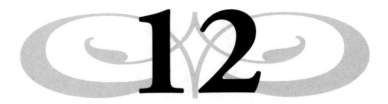

My doctor is busy. How do I get him or her to check my feet?

Take off your shoes and socks. If you have trouble doing this, ask the doctor's nurse or assistant to help you. Studies have shown that health care professionals are much more likely to examine the feet of a person with diabetes if the shoes and socks have already been removed when the health care provider comes into the examining room.

Another way to get your feet examined is to ask. Most health care professionals will readily check your feet whenever they are asked.

Finally, if you do not feel that you are getting enough attention to your feet from your primary physician, see your podiatrist or an orthopedic doctor who specializes in taking care of feet.

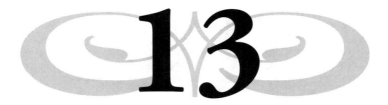

I cannot see my feet very well. How can I take care of them?

Sit down and pull your foot up on your knee or rest your foot on a footstool to get it closer to your eyes. Wear your glasses if you need to, and pick a place with good lighting. Use a mirror or magnifying mirror to examine the bottom of your feet. Medical supply stores and large drugstores have mirrors with long handles.

Be sure to run your hands over your feet. People with poor vision can learn what their feet feel like and can pick up changes in their feet by feeling them. If none of these suggestions work you might ask a friend or family member for help.

Do not cut your toenails if you cannot see well. Your health care provider, a nurse or assistant, or a home care nurse may be able to help you with foot care. Another option is to see a podiatrist. If you have good circulation and adequate feeling in your feet, your podiatrist may give you the OK to have pedicures done at a beauty salon or spa. If you do get a pedicure, it is often a good idea to take your own instruments with you to prevent the transmission of fungal or bacterial infections.

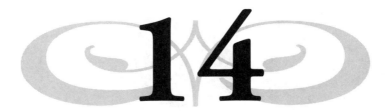

I cannot reach my feet very well. How can I take care of them every day?

Get a bath bench for your shower or tub in a drugstore or medical supply store. Have grab bars installed in your shower or tub. Get a long-handled bath brush or sponge on a handle, so you can wash your feet while sitting down or holding onto the grab bar. Rinse your feet before you stand up, because soapy feet are slippery.

You can leave one end of the towel on the floor and rub your foot over the towel to dry it. Dry as well as you can between the toes. You can also use the sponge on a handle to apply lotion to your feet, but you need two sponges: one for bathing and one for lotion. Keep the lotion sponge in a plastic bag.

Most people who have trouble reaching their feet wear slip-on shoes or shoes with Velcro fasteners. You can also try elastic laces, found in shoe repair shops. A long-handled shoehorn also comes in handy, as does a "sock-puller."

You might ask for a referral to an occupational therapist. An occupational therapist can help you find and use devices like sock-pullers and long-handled shoehorns. If flexibility is part of your problem, ask for help learning stretching exercises or yoga postures.

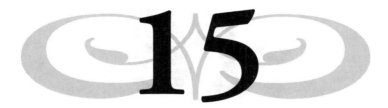

What changes in the foot are due to normal aging?

Changes can occur in our hardworking feet as we age, especially joint diseases like arthritis. Bones can shift out of position, rubbing against shoes and causing pain and the buildup of calluses or corns. We lose some of the fat pad that cushions the ball of the foot—and people with diabetes may lose it all—causing a callus to grow as a way to relieve the sharp pressure of bones on the soles of our feet. This and other changes can make us unsteady, and our gait or walking pattern may change. Our feet tend to get longer, wider, and flatter, which affects how our shoes fit.

You can offset some of the effects of aging. Always wear shoes that fit well. Sometimes changes in the shape of your feet occur so gradually that you do not notice how poorly your shoes fit, especially if you have nerve damage and cannot feel your feet. Don't wear shoes that you have saved for years for special occasions.

An unsteady gait can be a sign of another type of medical problem, so talk to your provider about it. It may just be time to get a cane. Your provider or physical therapist can give you tips on getting a cane of proper length and how to walk with it.

One of the best ways to keep your muscles, bones, and joints young is to stay active. This is also good for your diabetes. If you have never been active, you can begin by exercising sitting down.

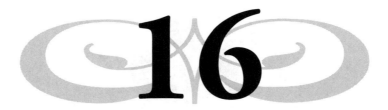

Does a meal plan have anything to do with my feet?

Yes. You know that achieving near-normal blood glucose levels can improve your chances of not having nerve damage or circulation problems. Part of managing your blood glucose is following a meal plan, along with exercising daily and taking diabetes medication if you need it.

What you eat affects your health, including your skin, muscles, and bones. A meal plan that is unbalanced, with too many processed foods (white flour, sugars, and fats) and too few vegetables and fruits, leaves you with fewer weapons to use against bacteria and fungus on the skin. Healthy eating for people with diabetes means eating the same healthy foods that everyone should eat. Especially important are the vitamins and the minerals that you can get from vegetables and fruits. You also want to be sure that you are getting enough calcium and magnesium for your bones. Ask for a referral to a registered dietitian (RD) if you need help designing or changing your meal plan to meet your needs and to manage your blood glucose levels.

What you eat also affects your blood fats and plays an important part in circulation and peripheral vascular disease (see pages 101–113).

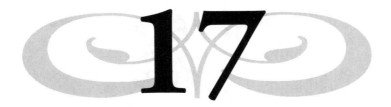

My providers have given me so many foot care instructions. Which ones do I really have to do?

The instructions you received will help you protect your feet—if you follow them. But most providers know that few people follow all the instructions all the time. If you miss a day or two of lubricating your dry skin, skip the prescribed antifungal gel for your athlete's foot one day, or forget to examine your feet one night, you'll probably be OK (no promises, however). But do try to follow your foot care plan, and remember these recommendations:

- Don't smoke. If you do and you're ready to quit, talk to your provider about getting help.
- Examine your feet daily.
- Don't use over-the-counter medications on your feet without consulting your health care provider.
- Don't go barefoot! Many minor injuries sustained while walking barefoot at home have been implicated in amputations.
- Wearing your special therapeutic shoes can prevent ulcers. In one study, patients who had healed ulcers were given therapeutic cushioned shoes with protective innersoles. Those who wore the shoes more than 60% of the time decreased their chances of getting another ulcer by 50% compared with those who wore them less time.
- Learn as much as you can about foot health. This book is a great place to start!

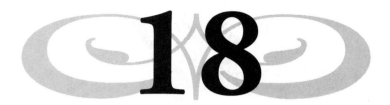

Does the American Diabetes Association have any foot care recommendations for people with diabetes?

Yes. The American Diabetes Association (ADA) develops and disseminates diabetes care standards, which are published annually. These statements represent the official position of the ADA. The ADA position statement on foot care, "Preventive Foot Care in People with Diabetes," can be found online at http://care.diabetesjournals.org/cgi/content/full/27/suppl_1/s63.

The foot care statement covers risk identification, foot exams, prevention of high-risk conditions, management of high-risk conditions, patient education, and provider education. Understanding how to prevent problems and what to do about them is crucial for diabetic foot care. This brief statement offers specific recommendations for people with diabetes as well as their care providers.

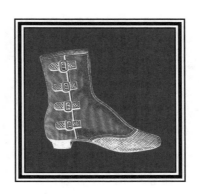

Chapter 2
Skin Care Tips

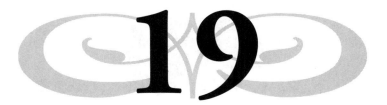

What is the best way for me to wash my feet?

The best way to wash your feet is in the bathtub or shower. Wash your feet just like you wash the rest of your body. If your feet have lost sensation due to neuropathy you may not be able to tell if the water is too hot. Check the temperature with your elbow, not with your toes! You can use any good soap. If you have dry skin, you might want to try soap with moisturizer to combat dryness. Soap that is not milled is more moisturizing. (Milling removes glycerin to make the soap harder and easier to shape.)

If you prefer, or if you have to, you can wash your feet in a pan of water. Take the same precautions and be sure that the water is not too hot. It is not necessary to buy a special footbath. If you cannot use the bathtub or shower, any plastic or metal tub the size of a dishpan will work. Don't soak your feet. This can dry out the skin excessively and even lead to infections. Be sure to rinse your feet well, and be sure to dry very well, especially between the toes. Use a soft fluffy towel to gently pat your feet dry. Don't rub.

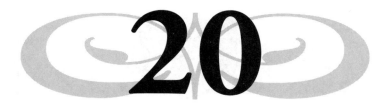

Why do I have such dry skin on my feet?

As we age, skin may become thinner and dryer, so your dry skin may be from normal aging. People tend to have more dry skin in winter because of heating systems blowing dry air. Bathing with very hot water or soaking can also contribute to dry skin because it washes away natural skin oils. Harsh soaps and detergents also remove these oils.

People with diabetes can get a type of nerve damage called autonomic neuropathy. The autonomic nerves control blood flow, sweating, and skin moisture. People who have autonomic neuropathy may notice that their feet sweat less or not at all. This can cause severe dry skin.

Several other problems can cause dry skin of the feet. If your dry skin problem is not helped by regularly using a hand or body lotion, seek the advice of your health care provider. In some cases prescription creams or lotions may be needed.

21

Do I need to use skin lotions? What kind should I use and how often?

Yes, you need to moisturize dry skin to prevent itching and cracking and to help keep germs out. Moisturizers are packaged as creams, lotions, ointments, and oils. For most people, any good body or hand lotion will do, as long as you remember to use it. Select a kind that you like and will actually use every day.

Avoid lotions with alcohol because it evaporates and takes moisture from the skin, which has a drying effect. Some people are sensitive to chemicals in highly perfumed or colored lotions, but there are lotions with no smell or color. Avoid lotions with lanolin if you are allergic to wool. Lotion with mineral oil may not work as well as lotions containing olive oil, almond oil, jojoba oil, or vegetable oils. Aloe vera gel is another good moisturizer.

Ask your health care provider or pharmacist to recommend a moisturizer. Products that contain lactic acid or urea help moisturize better than those with just emollients. You can get a prescription lotion if you have special problems or severe dry skin.

The best time to apply lotion is after a bath or a shower, to help seal in the moisture your body has absorbed. Do not apply moisturizers between your toes; these areas usually need no help in staying moist. Apply lotion one to three times a day. Keeping lotion in your sock drawer may help you remember to use it. If you prefer to apply lotion at bedtime, put on a pair of socks to keep the lotion off the sheets and help it soak in overnight.

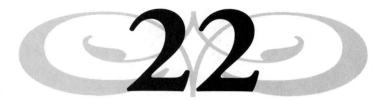

How can I tell whether I have athlete's foot fungus?

The only way to tell for sure is to have your health care provider examine it. He or she will take a small skin scraping and look at it under a microscope or try to grow it on a culture medium. However, when you have itchy, burning, red, soggy, flaky, or cracking skin or dry scales between your toes, it is most likely athlete's foot fungus. Many providers will treat these symptoms as athlete's foot fungus without actually testing for it.

Athlete's foot can also occur on the soles or sides of the feet with many of the same symptoms and problems. Often what looks like dry skin is really a fungal infection.

23

What should I do if I have athlete's foot fungus?

You can buy over-the-counter antifungal powders, sprays, and creams. Do not use harsh chemicals like chlorine bleach. Bleach does not kill the fungus and can burn your skin. Apply only a thin layer of medicine. When athlete's foot flares up, apply the medication at least twice a day (morning and night) for at least 4 weeks.

See your provider if you have redness, swelling, or a warm area anywhere on your foot, or if you see any pus. If you have fever or chills or your blood glucose levels are higher than usual, you may have an infection that needs to be treated.

Your provider can prescribe stronger antifungal creams and pills for severe cases of athlete's foot. Unfortunately, it may come back when treatment stops.

Remember to dry well between your toes. You can put on anti-fungal foot powder. Some people find that lacing a little lamb's wool between the toes helps keep that area dry. Don't use cotton balls or tissues because they stay moist and can pack down and increase pressure between the toes. Once you have treated the fungus on your feet you may need to disinfect your shoes and socks or buy new ones.

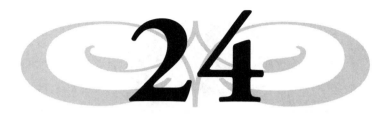

How can I prevent athlete's foot fungus?

There are several things you can do to prevent athlete's foot fungus from becoming a problem. The main one is to keep your feet clean and dry. Wear socks made of fibers that wick the moisture away from your skin. Cotton just stays moist. Put on a clean pair of socks every day. If your feet get wet during the day, change socks more often. Fungi thrive in dark, moist, warm areas.

Wear shoes with leather or fabric uppers that allow air to pass through. Allow your shoes to dry between wearings. If you have two pairs, alternate between them.

Avoid walking barefoot, especially in public areas such as pools, showers, and locker rooms. Even walking around your own house without protection may allow you to come in contact with fungi brought in on shoes from outside. Fungal infections are contagious. If you don't come in contact with the fungus, you won't catch it.

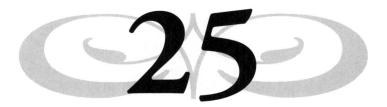

What should I do about foot odor?

Foot odor is caused by the breakdown of bacteria on the skin. Fungal infections of the skin and nails also may be the cause of the odor. Daily bathing, changing socks, and keeping the feet clean and dry can control this. Using an antibacterial soap and a soft brush to gently scrub away dead skin may help. If your feet get wet during the day, you will need to change socks more often.

Always wear socks when you wear shoes. Wear shoes that allow air to circulate, not plastic or synthetic shoes. Dry out your shoes between wearings. Some foot odor problems are related to smelly shoes rather than smelly feet. You may need to get new shoes.

If the problem continues, you might try an antiperspirant for feet or a foot powder designed to control foot odor. Special insoles with activated charcoal or silver and socks that are designed to help control foot odor are available.

Foot odor is sometimes a symptom of a serious problem such as a foot infection or foot ulcer that has gone undetected because of nerve damage. Inspect your feet carefully and if you detect a foot wound, see your provider immediately.

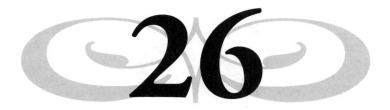

Why do my feet swell?

If both feet are swollen, it usually does not have much to do with your feet. If you have too much fluid in your system, it collects at the lowest part of the body due to gravity, and your feet and ankles swell. People with high blood pressure frequently have this kind of swelling. If your heart is too weak to pump blood around the body, the liquid parts of the blood tend to leak out of the blood vessels and collect in the lowest parts of the body. People with congestive heart failure have this kind of swelling. If your kidneys do not function well and you lose protein in your urine, your feet will swell.

Another cause of foot swelling is inactivity. When you are normally active during the day, the muscles in your legs help move blood and fluids back to the heart so they can recirculate. If you are sitting in a car or riding on an airplane all day, your leg muscles will not be working as much and fluid will pool in your feet and legs. That's why it's a good idea to get up and walk around every hour or two on an airplane or stop and walk around at a rest stop when you are in a car for long periods.

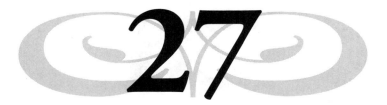

What should I do about foot swelling?

Elevate your feet and legs. Put your feet on a footstool, box, or another chair, or sit in a recliner with the footrest up. You can lie down on the couch and put your feet up on a pillow. Try to get your feet above the level of your heart. Any elevation is better than letting your feet hang down.

Another thing you can do is stay active. Remember, when you are walking, the force of your contracting leg muscles helps blood and fluids return to the heart and keeps them from pooling in your feet and legs.

In some cases, you may be asked to take diuretics, often called "water pills." Water pills make you urinate a lot and leave less fluid in the system. That is how they lower blood pressure and make less work for a weak heart to do. Take your water pills as directed. Most people find it best to take these pills first thing in the morning because they send you to the bathroom frequently. If you take them too close to bedtime, they might interrupt your sleep.

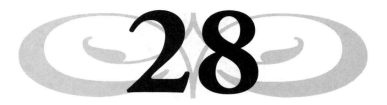

Should I wear support hose to control ankle swelling?

Ask your health care provider, because support hose should not be worn by people with poor circulation, skin disorders, infections, open wounds, or massive swelling. You must put them on before your feet or ankles swell, usually in the morning before you walk around much. Do not wear them to bed. Fluid will not accumulate in your feet while you are lying in bed.

Support hose come in several styles and colors for men and women and look like regular socks or stockings. Before buying below-the-knee support hose, measure around your calf at the widest part and from the floor to your knee. Do not guess. If you get the wrong size, they will be uncomfortable, and you will not wear them.

Your provider can advise you on how much "squeeze" you need. Hose come in different levels of compression—mild, moderate, and high. Some have high compression in the ankle and low compression in the calf. If they are too loose, they will not help, and if they are too tight, they cut off circulation. They can be custom knit to fit unusual leg shapes and fitted with zippers if you have trouble getting them on.

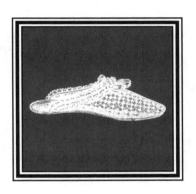

Chapter 3
Nail Care Tips

29

Can I cut my own toenails?

That depends on whether you can do it safely. If you have poor
circulation, or if your feet are numb from neuropathy, you should
not cut your own toenails. Many people have trouble cutting their
own toenails safely, especially if they are overweight or have
arthritis or vision problems. If you can see and reach your feet
well, if you have good nail clippers, and if you are careful, you can
trim your own toenails. You could use a large nail file or emery
board to file your nails. Filing is less risky than cutting. Nail files
for artificial fingernails are good for toenail filing because they
have coarser sandpaper than ordinary emery boards. If you have
nerve damage or poor circulation or you can't see or reach your
feet, ask for help.

You may have a family member or friend who is willing to help.
Another choice might be a beauty salon pedicure. You may want
to bring your own instruments to be sure you don't get bacterial
or fungal infections. Ask whether your provider has a nurse or
assistant to trim toenails. In some communities, foot care is available through senior center programs. Almost all podiatrists provide toenail care. Medicare or health insurance may pay all or part
of the cost for a podiatrist to trim your toenails if you have diabetes and meet certain criteria, such as having poor circulation.

30

What is the proper way to trim toenails when you have diabetes?

You may have seen instructions that say to cut your toenails straight across. However, this practice often leaves a sharp corner on the nail. It makes more sense to trim your nails with the contour of the toe, being sure all sharp edges are cut or filed smooth. The length of the toenail should be even with the end of the toe.

It is not a good idea to cut into the edges of the toenail or to try to treat ingrown toenails yourself. This sort of "bathroom surgery" is very risky for people with diabetes. If you do injure yourself, seek medical attention for any injury that does not heal promptly. If you have nerve damage or poor circulation and you cut yourself, see your provider right away. Do not wait until you develop an infection.

31

What is the best tool to use to trim my toenails?

Try the nail clippers that look like a pair of wire cutters or pliers. They are available in large drugstores, beauty supply houses, and cutlery stores. It is not necessary to have a sterile tool, but your toenail clippers should be kept clean, dry, and sharp. When you use a tool that is dull, you have to put more pressure on the clippers, and you can injure yourself if they slip.

Do not use pocketknives, kitchen knives, sewing scissors, or your teeth, or pick at your toenails with your fingers. Once you have diabetes, it is too risky to try to cut your toenails with anything except a good pair of toenail clippers.

It is advisable not to share clippers with others. Fungal infections are contagious and may be passed from person to person.

32

What should I do if I nick myself while trimming my toenails?

If you have nerve damage or poor circulation, see your health care provider. If you don't, wash the injury with soap and water and pat it dry. It is generally not necessary to apply antiseptic creams to the wound. You may apply a bandage to keep it clean, but do not wrap the bandage tightly. Make it loose enough so that the circulation is not cut off if the toe or foot swells.

Do not be reassured if the wound does not hurt, because nerve damage may prevent you from feeling it. A wound that does not hurt may still be a serious injury.

Change the bandage and inspect the wound every day. Ask for help if you are having trouble seeing or caring for the injury. If you notice any redness, swelling, pus, or an area of increased warmth on your foot, or if the foot does not heal in a reasonable amount of time, report it to your health care provider right away. If you have an infection, you may need to take an oral antibiotic to cure it.

33

What should I do if I have very thick toenails?

A thick toenail can put lots of pressure on the toe and cause an ulcer, so it is a good idea to have it trimmed down or removed. Whether or not you can trim it yourself depends on how thick it is. Most people need help. It is best to go to a podiatrist or health care provider who is trained to trim thick nails and has special tools to do the job.

A fungus usually causes thick toenails. Creams, oils, and liquid drops are sold over-the-counter to treat fungal toenails. While these may help soften the nail and retard the fungus somewhat, they usually do not make it go away. The first step is to see if a fungus is really causing the problem. Your doctor will take a sample of the nail either for microscopic examination or for a culture.

There are prescription pills that may eliminate the fungus on your toenails. Because these medications can affect the liver, you will need to have a blood test before you start the medicine and another one about 6 weeks into the 3-month treatment. If you want to cure fungal toenails, talk with your provider about these pills. They can cost hundreds of dollars, so be sure to discuss the costs involved. Be aware that the fungus might return after you stop taking the medication. You should talk to your doctor about what you can do to minimize the possibility of the fungus coming back. In severe or recurrent cases, your doctor may suggest removing the nail and the root of the nail to prevent regrowth.

34

What should I do if I have ingrown toenails?

Ingrown toenails are a common problem for people who have diabetes—and for those who don't. This painful condition results when the nail grows into the skin. You're more likely to get it if you trim the toenails too short and cut down the sides of the toenail. Trim your toenails a bit longer, following the curve of the toe without leaving any sharp corners. If the toenail grows into the skin, it breaks the skin, and infection may develop. If the nail has simply been cut incorrectly, a podiatrist or other health care provider can remove the ingrown portion. If you have nerve damage, the ingrown toenail may not hurt, but it certainly needs professional care.

If the problem comes back, the podiatrist will numb the toe and remove a corner of the nail. Sometimes a chemical is put into the corner to kill the root and keep the ingrown portion from coming back. Fixing the problem permanently will not only prevent future pain but also may eliminate the possibility of infection. This is especially important for people with diabetes.

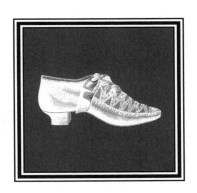

Chapter 4
Shoes and Socks Tips

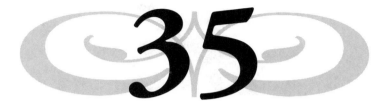

What are the best shoes to wear when you have diabetes?

A lace-up shoe with a high, rounded toe box is ideal. The upper part of the shoe should be a soft, breathable material such as leather or fabric instead of plastic or synthetic materials. Avoid sandals, clogs, thongs, or flip-flops, because they do not provide the same protection that a closed shoe does. If you have a callus or deformity, you need a shoe with a soft innersole that redistributes the pressure on the sole of your foot. With a bunion or hammertoe, you may need extra-width or extra-depth shoes.

If you have trouble tying laces, try shoes with Velcro fasteners. Most tied shoes can be converted to Velcro fasteners at a shoe repair shop. Elastic shoelaces allow you to get your shoes off and on without untying the laces.

Avoid tight, pointed shoes. High heels are not good for any foot—especially one with diabetes. They force the entire weight of the body onto the front of the foot, changing the shape, greatly increasing pressure, and causing ulcers. Look for a shoe that is shaped like a foot. While this sounds reasonable, it can be a challenging task, especially for women. A pedorthist (certified shoe fitter) can help you pick the right shoe. It's worth the effort. Good-quality athletic shoes or walking shoes are often excellent choices as well.

36

I've been told that people with diabetes should wear shoes all the time. I have wall-to-wall carpeting, and I like to go barefoot in my home. Should I?

No. Carpeting does not prevent you from stepping on pins, tacks, toys, dog bones, and whatever the cat brought in. Doctors often remove small pieces of glass, wood splinters, and even needles from dropped insulin syringes from the feet of people who have walked without shoes at home. Over 80% of amputations can be traced back to a minor traumatic event!

Most people do not take their shoes off before they enter their homes. The shoes track in viruses, fungi, and bacteria, which are deposited on floor surfaces. Viruses can cause warts, fungi can cause athlete's foot and nail diseases, and bacteria can cause infections. If you walk barefoot in your home, you may come in contact with these disease-producing organisms.

Make it a habit to protect your feet at all times—at the beach or pool (water shoes), in public showers (shower shoes), and even in your own home (house shoes or slippers). The only time to go without shoes is when you are in bed or bathing.

37

How can I tell whether my shoes fit?

One way is to purchase them from a podiatrist (foot specialist) or a trained shoe fitter (pedorthist). Have both feet measured every time you buy shoes, and shop for shoes in the afternoon or evening when your feet may be swollen. Your shoes need to fit all day. When you try on shoes, check that the ball of the foot rests in the widest part of the shoe. Walk a few steps and look for signs of a poor fit, such as the foot rolling over the sole or too much space between the heel and the back of the shoe. Notice whether the shoe bends where your foot does, and be sure there is plenty of room for your toes. There should be a half-inch space between the longest toe and the end of the toe box, but the shoes should not slip. (The longest toe is not always the big toe.) Be sure the toe box is high enough and does not press on your toes.

If you have foot deformities or have had an ulcer that is now healed, you should have shoes prescribed and fitted or custom-made by a podiatrist, orthopedic surgeon, or pedorthist. If you have nerve damage, even your properly fitted new shoes may feel too big. Also remember that people's feet tend to get longer, wider, and flatter as the years go by. You will not always wear the same size.

38

My feet are different sizes. Do I have to buy two pairs of shoes?

It is very common for one foot to be slightly larger or wider than the other. If you need two different-sized shoes or if you have only one foot, you might want to contact the National Odd Shoe Exchange (www.oddshoe.org) or the One Shoe Crew (sally_tvarez@hotmail.com). These organizations help their members with mismatched or odd-sized feet to find shoes. Some members are matched with another member who has exactly the opposite shoe size problem so that they can share shoe purchases rather than having to buy two different-sized pairs to come up with one wearable pair. These groups are also of value to people with amputations who may need only one shoe.

39

Why should I inspect my shoes every day, and what am I looking for?

You are looking for anything that might injure your feet, especially if you have lost feeling in them. Look over the top and sole of the shoe, shake it out, and run your hand into it. Look and feel for any pebbles or other foreign objects, and check for nails or tacks that may be coming through the sole. Look for cracked uppers or rough seams that could rub a blister. Replace shoes with worn or loose linings. If heels or soles are worn down, get new shoes or have them resoled so your foot is getting the support it needs. If your podiatrist has prescribed special insoles or orthotics, periodically pull these out and check them as well. The soft inserts that often come with therapeutic shoes flatten out and must be replaced three times a year.

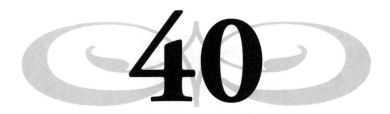

What are the best socks to wear?

Socks or stockings should be made from acrylic or synthetic material such as Cool Max that wicks moisture away from your skin. They should not be too tight or too loose and should fit without folds or wrinkles. Choose socks without seams. Garters or socks that bind may cut off circulation to your feet and legs. If the elastic at the top of your socks is too tight, cut a notch into the cuff of the sock.

Socks shaped like feet are preferable to tube socks, which tend to thin out over the heel and bunch up in the front. Change into clean socks daily. Throw away socks with holes. Repaired socks may have rough patches that can irritate your foot.

You can find extra large socks in big and tall shops, athletic stores, and department stores. Sports stores may have socks that are double knit on the bottom to provide an extra layer of cushioning. Just be sure that they don't make your shoes too tight. When you are purchasing new shoes, try them on with socks of the thickness that you will be wearing.

Wear nylon stockings or panty hose for the shortest time possible. Nylon is not a breathable fabric (that's why they make raincoats out of it!), so change into some socks as soon as you can.

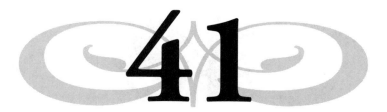

Does sock color matter? I've always thought white socks were best.

Sock color is generally irrelevant. Some people, however, are allergic to the dye in some socks and, therefore, wear white socks. If you do not have an allergy to the dye, you may wear any color you choose.

Some people with diabetic neuropathy and insensitive feet also wear white socks. Wearing white helps them see blood or drainage on their socks if they get a cut or a sore on their feet. Daily foot exams, which are recommended for everyone with diabetes, should eliminate the need to depend on sock stains to tell if there is a foot wound.

Some new materials also may change the color of your socks. Several companies now incorporate silver within the fabric. Silver in socks is said to kill bacteria and fungi, making for a healthier foot environment.

42

Do I need custom shoes?

Most people with diabetes do not need custom-made shoes.
Custom-made shoes are necessary only for people with significant
deformities that cannot be accommodated by a stock shoe.
However, if you are at risk for ulceration or amputation, you may
need special, therapeutic shoes—for example, ones with extra
depth and inserts. You are considered to be at risk if you have
already had a toe or partial-foot amputation, if you have a foot
deformity, if you have ever had an ulcer that is now healed, or if
you have diabetes-related foot problems such as poor circulation
(peripheral vascular disease) or nerve damage (diabetic neuropathy). A podiatrist or other health care provider who can examine
your feet is the best person to advise you about custom shoes.

43

Will Medicare pay for my therapeutic shoes?

Prescription footwear can help prevent some foot problems. Medicare pays for therapeutic footwear when you meet certain criteria and have your diabetes care provider complete the proper form. This benefit covers custom-molded shoes, extra-depth shoes, inserts, and some shoe modifications. Your physician must certify on the form that you are in a diabetes care plan, have evidence of foot disease, and need therapeutic footwear. You can get the form from prescription shoe stores, Medicare, or your podiatrist or diabetes care provider. Often, the podiatrist or pedorthist will help you get the forms completed by your diabetes care provider.

A podiatrist writes the prescription for the therapeutic shoes, and a podiatrist or pedorthist supplies them. You must buy the footwear from a qualified supplier. Some suppliers require you to pay for the shoes and inserts and then get reimbursed by Medicare; others will wait for Medicare to pay for them directly, so that you do not have to lay out the money. In either case, Medicare covers 80% of the allowed amount and you, or your secondary insurance if you have any, must pay the balance. Suppliers who participate in Medicare cannot charge more than Medicare allows. Suppliers who do not accept Medicare assignment may charge more than Medicare allows, and you must pay the difference.

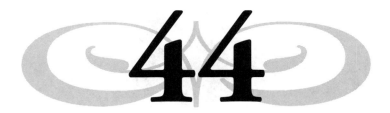

Do I need special insoles for my shoes?

Maybe. You can relieve pressure on the soles of your feet by wearing a cushioning layer between your foot and the floor. If you wear thin-soled shoes or if you have high-pressure areas on your feet, it is a good idea to add insoles to your shoes. High-pressure areas are where calluses develop. Most ulcers begin under a callus. If you can prevent or reduce the size of a callus, you may prevent an ulcer from developing in that area, too.

Some insoles are available in drugstores, grocery stores, sporting goods stores, and running shoe stores for less than $10 a pair. Running shoe stores also have insoles with extra arch support for $15 to $30. Be sure to check with your foot care specialist before buying any insole. An insole will raise your foot in the shoe, so be sure that you have plenty of room in the toe of the shoes. If your shoes are too tight with the insoles, you would do better with half-insoles that do not go under the toes. Many insole materials lose their cushioning effect and will need replacement every 3 to 4 months.

If you have foot deformities or large calluses on your feet, you may need orthotics, which are inserts that are specially made to fit your feet (see page 53).

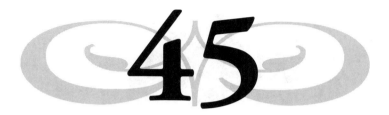

What are orthotics?

Orthotics are specially designed insoles that are worn inside your shoes to control the way your foot moves or to support painful or at-risk areas of the foot. Often mistakenly called arch supports, they can do much more than that. Additions, top covers, extensions, or wedges can be added to the orthotics to hold your feet in a more stable position inside the shoe. This can help you walk normally, relieve foot pain, avoid calluses and corns, and even help with knee, hip, and lower back pain.

Orthotics are usually custom-made using a plaster model of your foot. They may be made of a rigid material, like plastic, but can also be made of leather or other soft materials. Graphite orthotics are durable and can be made very thin for comfort. Properly made orthotics should be comfortable. Orthotics should always be prescribed by a foot care specialist. Never buy these devices through the mail or from stores without a prescription.

Orthotics can be expensive, so check to see whether your health plan will help you pay for them. Often they will be covered. One pair may not fit inside all your shoes, so you may want separate orthotics for dress shoes or sports. Orthotics must be replaced periodically, so ask the person who made them when you'll need new ones.

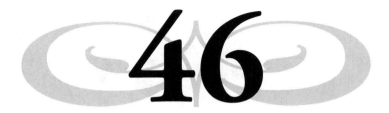

What is a pedorthist, and do I need to see one?

A pedorthist is a professional shoe fitter who has been trained in both foot anatomy and shoe construction. Pedorthists fill prescriptions for footwear and orthotics. A custom shoe store may have a pedorthist on staff. A nationally certified pedorthist may use the initials "C Ped" after his or her name.

If you have a severe foot deformity, you are probably already familiar with people trained in this specialty. If you have trouble getting shoes that fit properly or you need special adjustments to your shoes because your feet are changing shape or you're losing feeling in your feet, it might be a good idea to see a pedorthist.

Before you see a pedorthist, however, an exam by a foot specialist is recommended. Only a doctor can make a diagnosis and prescribe the appropriate footwear and modifications that you may need.

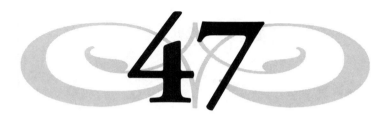

I have had a partial foot amputation. Can I just put padding in my shoes and continue to wear the shoes I wore before the surgery?

Maybe. You need to have your foot examined by a podiatrist or an orthopedic surgeon to see where the pressure points are and whether there are any new ones since the surgery. An amputation "creates" a foot deformity, and it is important for your shoes to fit properly so that they do not rub a blister or cause a buildup of callus. You may need orthotics or a specially made shoe. Your doctor may also want to add material to the shoe insert to fill in the empty space and prevent shifting of the foot or abnormal pressure spots.

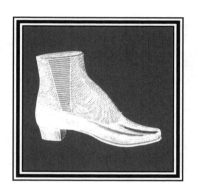

Chapter 5
Treating Minor
Problems

48

I have a blister on my foot. What should I do?

If you have neuropathy or poor circulation, see your health care provider immediately! Don't wait until it gets infected. Then the first thing to do is to stop wearing the offending shoe. Wash the area with warm water and mild soap and dry well. Do not break the blister—this can allow germs to get under the skin. Cover the blister with a dry bandage. If the blister breaks, leave the loose skin as a covering over the wound until it heals. It is not necessary to apply antiseptics, antibiotic ointments, or chemicals to the blister.

Inspect the blistered area daily. If there is redness, tenderness, swelling, pus, or a warm area around the wound after the first day, you may be getting an infection. See your provider to get antibiotics. Over-the-counter antibiotic creams are not strong enough to treat a foot infection in a person with diabetes. If the wound is deep, gets larger, or does not heal within a few days, have it checked immediately.

Don't wear the shoes again until the blister is entirely healed. You might need extra padding, different socks, or something else to keep them from rubbing. Wear the shoes for a short while; then check your feet for signs of another blister. It is better to throw them away than to continue wearing shoes that injure your feet.

49

I stubbed my toe. What should I do?

Well, that depends on how much you have injured it. While a stubbed toe can be excruciatingly painful, the actual injury can vary from minor to severe. If you don't have peripheral vascular disease, put ice on the injury and elevate it higher than your heart to relieve the swelling and pain. Is the toe in an abnormal position? Do you have continued pain, swelling, or an inability to put weight on the foot? If so, you need to see your health care provider for an X-ray of your foot to make sure that you have not broken any bones. If you neglect a fracture, particularly of the big toe, it can result in a painful deformity. You need early treatment to prevent a deformity from occurring. Sometimes people with nerve damage do not feel pain and can injure a foot or toe quite severely without knowing it. If you have nerve damage, check your feet carefully with your eyes and your hands after any injury to see how bad it is.

If blood accumulates under the toenail, it can put pressure on the toe. You may need to visit your health care provider to have the pressure relieved. Do not try to relieve it yourself by puncturing the nail or performing any other home surgery. When you have diabetes, it is best to have a health care provider treat all foot injuries.

50

I stepped on a nail. What should I do?

See your health care provider right away. Puncture wounds are a serious matter, especially when you have diabetes. Nails and other sharp objects do not have to be rusty to cause lockjaw (tetanus) or to cause an infection in your foot. Punctures through shoes are especially dangerous because a little rubber from the sole of the shoe sometimes enters the wound and causes an especially nasty type of infection.

Wash the area with warm water and mild soap and dry well. Cover the wound with a dry bandage. It is not necessary to apply antiseptics or antibiotic ointments. Keep the area covered until you can see your doctor and receive appropriate care and instructions. All adults should have tetanus booster shots repeated at least every 10 years. If you are not sure when you had your last tetanus booster, it is safe to have another one when you are injured.

51

My toenail fell off. What should I do?

After a toenail injury, it is not uncommon for the nail to fall off. Sometimes this happens with very thick fungal nails. Toenails grow slowly—much more slowly than fingernails. It will usually grow back within 12–18 months. Keep the area clean and dry while waiting for the new nail to grow back. Protect it from any further damage by not going barefoot and by wearing shoes that have plenty of room for your toes. The nail-growing cells may have been damaged during the injury, so sometimes the new toenail will be a different shape.

Remember, if you have circulation problems, any foot injury should be checked by your foot specialist.

52

Can I use over-the-counter corn and callus removers?

No, you really should not use these products if you have diabetes. Usually the product label will say, "Not for use by people with diabetes." Corn and callus removers, corn plasters, and similar products are harsh chemicals, usually acids. They decrease the buildup of hard skin by softening and burning away the corn or callus. If you have diabetic nerve damage, you might not be able to feel it if the chemicals burned too much or got on the surrounding normal skin. It is dangerous for a person with diabetes to get any breaks in the skin because of the risks of infection and difficulty with healing. Therefore, you should avoid putting harsh chemicals on your feet.

Whenever possible, you should treat the cause of the problem so that corns and calluses do not form. These products just try to remove the hard skin. See your podiatrist if you have a corn or callus that needs to be treated.

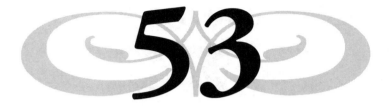

What should I do about a corn between my toes?

Corns between the toes that touch each other are called soft corns or kissing corns. Bones in adjacent toes rubbing together cause these corns. Shoes that squeeze the toes together aggravate soft corns. Sometimes they are very painful.

You can change shoes, add padding, and have surgery for soft corns. Switch to shoes that have a soft and high rounded toe box that does not press your toes together. You can buy special toe separator pads made of silicone or soft foam rubber, or you can loosely lace some lamb's wool between the toes to decrease the rubbing. Do not use cotton or tissues between the toes because these materials can pack down and actually increase the pressure. Inspect your feet every day, including between the toes. See your podiatrist or another health care provider if you think the soft corn needs to be trimmed, or if it is irritated or ulcerated.

Surgery to correct the problem causing the corn is often the best solution to prevent the corn from occurring. Elective foot surgery is often more important for people with diabetes than for the general population. Many foot ulcers begin as a callus or corn, so preventing the corn can prevent ulcers, infections, and amputations.

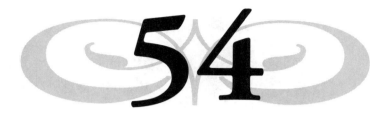

What should I do about a callus on the bottom of my foot?

Try to decrease the high pressure on that spot by wearing shoes with a soft insole and a cushioned outer sole. Don't wear house shoes with little cushioning or go barefoot, because this will make the callus worse. A hard callus is like having a rock in your shoe. Most foot ulcers occur in the damaged tissue beneath a callus. You need to be evaluated by a foot care professional to see what is causing the callus.

To deal with a callus, you can change shoes, get orthotics, moisturize the skin, trim the callus, or have surgery. Moisturizing the callused area with a good lotion will help keep it soft. A callus can be carefully sanded down with an emery board, callus file, or a pumice stone. It may be easier to remove after a bath or shower when the skin is still soft. Go easy and do not injure yourself by scrubbing too hard. Buff the area a little every other day instead of trying to remove the callus all at once. Never try to remove a callus by cutting or trimming it with a razor blade. See your podiatrist or health care provider for ongoing callus care.

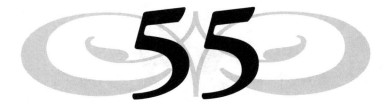

What should I do about a wart on the bottom of my foot?

The word "plantar" means the bottom of the foot, so plantar warts are just warts that are located there. Plantar warts are caused by the papilloma virus, which gets under the skin. In some people, the warts disappear without any treatment. In others, plantar warts hang around for years even when they are treated. People with diabetes should always seek treatment.

Although there are many home remedies for plantar warts, the best solution is to see your health care provider or podiatrist. If left alone, a wart may spread into multiple warts that can cover large areas of the foot. Since they are caused by a virus, they are contagious and can be spread to family members. Sometimes it is difficult even for professionals to tell the difference between a plantar wart and a callus. There are several treatments for plantar warts. They can be trimmed, padded, or removed with chemicals; burned with liquid nitrogen; or removed by surgery. It is important not to leave a painful scar on the bottom of the foot that can affect walking, so it is best not to try any of these treatments by yourself.

56

What is a bunion? What should I do if I have one?

A bunion is a deformity in the joint of the big toe that causes the toe to point away from the arch instead of straight ahead. There is usually an unsightly bump on the inside of the foot. It is believed that uneven weight distribution during walking and stresses in the joints cause bunions and that they tend to run in families. Wearing shoes with pointed toes probably contributes to developing bunions.

If you have a painful bunion or it is difficult to get your shoes to fit, discuss what to do with your foot doctor. Don't put it off. You may need special shoes, orthotics, or padding. Deformities like bunions are a major risk factor for ulcers and amputation. Early surgery is often the best treatment for people with diabetes. Modern bunion surgery not only removes the bump but also attempts to correct the mechanical problem that caused it so that the bunion does not grow back. Severe bunions that have been there for years may even require joint replacement surgery, similar to replacing an arthritic knee joint. Bunion surgery can take about 6 weeks to heal, so you will want to have your blood glucose levels as close to normal as possible before and after the surgery to encourage healing.

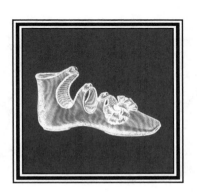

Chapter 6
Exercise Tips

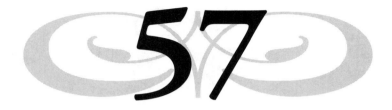

What foot precautions should I follow when walking, running, or jogging?

Have a thorough foot exam to discover any deformity, lack of feeling, or poor circulation. Wear socks with good cushioning that are made from a material such as acrylic or CoolMax. Good-quality walking or running shoes may prevent injury. Always take the time to warm up. Cool down and stretch after the exercise activity and inspect your feet for redness, blisters, or hot spots. If you have pain during exercise, stop and try to figure out what is wrong. You may need orthotics to help your feet work normally during physical activity—especially if you are active and have knee pain or pain in the arch or heel area of your foot (plantar fasciitis).

If you have a loss of feeling in your feet, limit repetitive weight-bearing exercises such as jogging and using stair-climbers because of the high pressure on your feet and possible injury that you wouldn't be able to feel. Do not do weight-bearing exercises when you have a foot ulcer. When the ulcer has healed, make sure to ask your doctor what caused it and take special precautions when exercising to keep it from coming back.

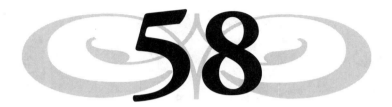

What forms of exercise are good for people with diabetic foot complications?

Walking can actually improve circulation in your legs and feet by forcing the blood vessels to work harder and expand. In fact, this is the recommended exercise for people with intermittent claudication (pain in the calf due to poor circulation). Walking is good for your heart and for your diabetes management, too. Try to walk for 30 to 60 minutes every day. Can't do it all at once? Try two 15- to 20-minute walks.

If you have lost much of the feeling in your feet, you can participate in non-weight-bearing exercises, such as swimming, bicycling, or rowing; upper-body exercises, such as weight lifting; and range of motion and stretching exercises. You can do yoga. You will achieve your best level of fitness if you do several different types of exercise during the week. For example, you can do stretching exercises one day and strength-building exercises the next day. Aerobic exercise (e.g., walking, running, biking, swimming) should be performed every day. If you row or bicycle on a machine, take care that the foot straps don't injure your feet. In a pool, you should wear aqua shoes to protect your feet.

Remember that your household chores, such as vacuuming and gardening, count as exercise, too.

59

Should I wear special shoes when exercising?

Yes, you should always wear good-quality athletic shoes that are made for the activity you are doing. This means wearing running shoes for running, golfing shoes for golfing, and bowling shoes for bowling. Almost every sport is associated with a special type of shoe appropriate to the particular activity. These shoes are important for preventing injury. And they may help you perform better and enjoy the sport more! If you are in doubt about which shoes to wear, a good running shoe, such as the kind used for running marathons, offers support and stability to protect your feet from injury. Be sure to buy your shoes from a knowledgeable salesperson.

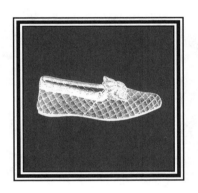

Chapter 7
Identifying Major Problems

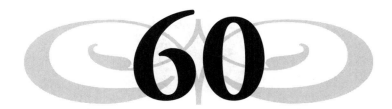

Is there a quick way for me to determine my risk for serious foot problems related to my diabetes?

You can ask your health care provider to check your feet. If you have pulses present in your feet, good sensation, no foot deformities, and no history of foot ulcer or amputation, you can assume you are in a low-risk category.

If, however, you have poor circulation, loss of sensation, a foot deformity (such as a bunion or hammertoe), or a history of a previous foot ulcer, or you have had part of a foot amputated, you are a high-risk patient. If you have more than one of these problems, your risk for future trouble increases drastically, and you need to take extra precautions.

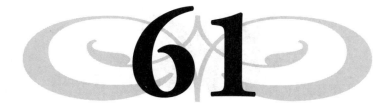

61

How do I know when I have a foot ulcer?

A foot ulcer is an open sore somewhere on your foot. The term "ulcer" refers to a wound or hole in the skin. We often hear about a stomach ulcer, which is a hole in the lining of the stomach. A foot ulcer is a break in the skin that is usually, but not always, shaped like a crater. Foot ulcers often occur in high-pressure areas, so it is common to find one under a callus or surrounded by callus. The most common foot ulcer locations are on the bottom or side of the big toe and on the ball of the foot, especially under the big toe joint. The ball of the foot under the little toe joint is also a common place for foot ulcers. However, diabetic foot ulcers can occur anywhere on the feet. Be aware that the actual break in the skin can be very small, but a larger ulcer may be hidden from view under the surrounding callus or skin. This is why it is important to have your feet inspected by a professional if you think you might have a foot ulcer. Most amputations are preceded by a foot ulcer. Treatment of ulcers is, therefore, of vital importance.

The only way for you to know whether you have a foot ulcer is by seeing it or feeling it. That is why people with diabetes should inspect their feet carefully every day.

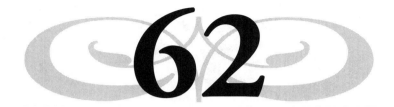

How do I avoid getting foot ulcers?

You can take several very important steps to protect your feet. Keep your blood glucose levels as close to normal as you can. Inspect your feet every day and after exercising. Get regular medical attention for your feet at least several times a year. Many ulcers are preceded by calluses, so be sure you see a foot doctor and treat these calluses aggressively. There is no magic to avoiding foot complications. The key is to develop a routine that includes commonsense, everyday attention to your feet.

- Keep your feet clean and dry.
- Wear well-fitting shoes and socks.
- Don't go barefoot.
- Don't soak your feet.
- Don't put lotion between your toes, but put it on the rest of your foot.
- Get monofilament testing at least once a year.
- Treat calluses aggressively by seeing a foot care specialist.
- Get any injury to your foot seen right away!

What should I do if I get a foot ulcer?

Have any foot ulcer examined by a health care professional immediately. Once you have received treatment, the wound should begin to heal in a week or two. Complete healing, however, may take quite some time. You must follow the treatment plan exactly as prescribed by your foot specialist. Usually, the doctor will trim or cut away (debride) the dead tissue, apply a dressing, and, if the wound is infected, prescribe antibiotics. There are many dressing materials that may help heal your wound. It is likely that you will be asked to change your shoes. You must not walk on an ulcer without protection. Use bed rest, crutches, or a wheelchair, but stay off that foot.

If the wound is not improving after a week or two, your doctor will change the treatment plan. Be sure that you are doing all you can to follow the plan and help your foot to heal.

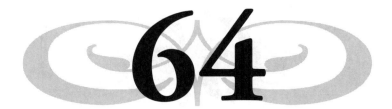

This foot ulcer is not getting better. What should I do?

If you are following the care plan and not walking on the ulcer but it still isn't healing, your podiatrist will certainly change the treatment plan. There are many new wound treatments that promote healing. Artificial skin products may be used to cover the hole while it heals. Extra oxygen to the wound, either pumped into a boot at home or applied under pressure often in a hyperbaric oxygen tank, can stimulate healing. A vascular surgeon may need to evaluate the ulcer to determine whether surgery might restore circulation to the foot and help heal the ulcer. You may also need a nutritional consultation to make sure your intake of protein, vitamins, and minerals is adequate for optimal healing. If a bony protrusion is causing the ulcer, surgery may be needed to change the position of the bone or remove it. Although surgery is not pleasant, it can be necessary to save a limb.

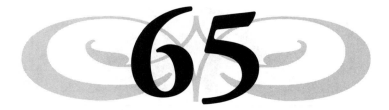

How do I know whether I have an infection?

Some signs of infection are

- redness
- swelling
- increased warmth
- pain, tenderness, or limited motion of the affected part
- pus or drainage from the wound

If you have one or two of these signs, have your health care provider check your wound as soon as possible to determine whether you have an infection.

Other signs that an infection has spread beyond the wound are fever, chills, or unusually high blood glucose levels. If you have any of these signs, you need to be seen immediately and should go at once to an emergency room if your regular health care provider cannot see you right away.

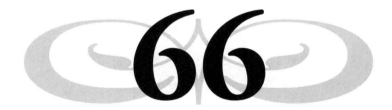

66

I had a foot ulcer that is now healed. What can I do to prevent another ulcer from forming?

Having a history of a previous foot ulcer is the greatest risk factor for getting another ulcer. About 70% of people who have a healed ulcer get another ulcer within 5 years. Since an ulcer precedes most amputations, prevention is very important.

Primarily, you should closely follow the instructions of your podiatrist. He or she will want to see you frequently to monitor your foot health. If the cause of the original ulcer is known, it should be corrected if possible, even if it involves bone surgery. Pressure relief is very important, and you will probably need special insoles or shoes to protect your feet. They should be worn all the time. Many insurance companies, including Medicare, will help pay for these shoes and inserts.

If you have calluses, your doctor must trim them regularly. Calluses increase pressure and often precede an ulcer. Never trim them yourself or use callus removers.

Inspect your feet at least once a day. If necessary, use a mirror to see the bottom of your feet or have a family member help you. If you notice any changes, such as a break in the skin or increased redness or warmth, notify your doctor at once.

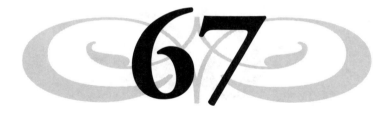

I have had a number of foot infections, one requiring removal of bone. Are there any new treatments for foot infections?

New medications and treatments are constantly becoming available. For example, until recently, bacteria that were resistant to many antibiotics had to be treated by long-term intravenous medications. Now there are oral antibiotics that work just as well, or better, than these intravenous drugs to treat diabetic foot infections and infections caused by resistant germs. But bacteria can develop resistance to new medications as well, so they must be used wisely.

Diabetic foot infections may also be treated by the application of oxygen, either topically or under pressure (hyperbaric oxygen). Some foot surgeons mix antibiotics into a kind of bead that is placed in an infected wound to kill the bacteria directly. Silver also kills bacteria, and many wound dressings now contain silver. In addition, open wounds may benefit from the application of suction through a vacuum system.

Keeping up with new technologies is a never-ending learning process. Of course, doctors who treat infections and wounds don't rely solely on new therapies. Tried-and-true wound treatments are still the basis for healing most infections.

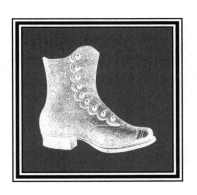

Chapter 8
Complications—
Nerve Damage

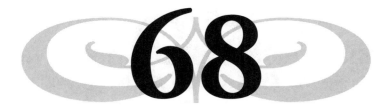

What is peripheral neuropathy?

Peripheral neuropathy is the name for damage to sensory, motor, and autonomic nerves. Motor and sensory nerves help you move and feel the world around you. In the feet, autonomic nerves control perspiration. "Peripheral" means at the edges or away from the center. In this case, the feet are farthest from the center of the body. "Neuro" means nerves and "pathy" means "a disorder of." Because the longest nerves are usually affected first, symptoms such as tingling, burning, or numbness appear first in the feet and hands.

You can think of the nervous system as being like the electrical system in your house. The wires to the lights and appliances are the peripheral nerves, and the fuse box and the main electric cable are the central nervous system (the brain and spinal cord).

When motor nerves are damaged, muscles in your foot can become weak and allow the shape of the foot to change. Toes can curl up, and the fat pad on the bottom of the foot can shift so that it no longer protects the skin on the bottom of the foot. Bones can get very close to the skin and can cause calluses. The sensory nerve damage prevents you from feeling pain, so a callus can become an ulcer without your knowing it. Autonomic nerve problems can cause dryness of the skin.

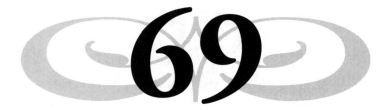

How does diabetes cause nerve damage?

Nobody really knows. It is pretty certain that higher than normal blood glucose levels are part of the cause. We do know that keeping your blood glucose levels close to normal can lower your chances of getting neuropathy, that people with high blood glucose levels are more likely to have neuropathy, and that the longer a person has diabetes, the more likely he or she is to have neuropathy.

There are several theories about how blood glucose levels affect nerves. It is possible that glucose coats the proteins in the nerves and that the glucose-coated proteins no longer function normally. Or it might be that high blood glucose levels interfere with chemical events in the nerves. High blood glucose levels may damage the insulation layer of cells around the nerves. Or they may damage the tiny blood vessels that supply the nerves, so that the nerves do not get enough oxygen and nutrients.

Researchers are working to understand the causes of neuropathy and to find treatments to avoid the damage that it does.

70

How do I know whether I have peripheral neuropathy?

If you have had diabetes for more than 10 years and you have not kept your blood glucose levels close to normal, you likely have some symptoms of nerve damage. It affects as many as 75% of all people with diabetes. Do you have muscle weakness, cramps, and feelings in your feet and legs such as numbness, tingling, pins and needles, and burning sensations? Do your feet bother you more at night? Have you had any episodes of fainting or vomiting or had a change in bowel habits, bladder control, or sexual functioning? These systems can be affected by diabetic nerve damage too.

Although there is no one specific test that all doctors use to check for neuropathy, there are some that are widely accepted. Your doctor may touch your feet with a small, thin fiber called a monofilament. If you can't feel this light touch, you have lost sensation. Similarly, you should be able to feel the vibrations of a tuning fork on your feet. A nerve conduction study, which tests the speed of electrical transmission through the nerves, may also be used.

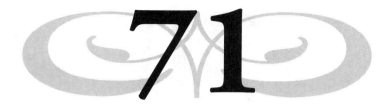

Can peripheral neuropathy cause foot deformities?

Yes. Three types of neuropathy are associated with diabetes: autonomic, sensory, and motor. In the feet, autonomic neuropathy affects perspiration and the dryness of the skin. Although this dryness can be a problem, it does not change the shape of the feet.

Sensory neuropathy affects how the feet feel. This type of neuropathy causes numbness and/or pain. If your feet are numb, you often will not feel pain, and you may walk on a foot that is being damaged. A Charcot foot is a breakdown of the structure of the foot—multiple fractures and a destruction of the bony architecture. The arch area may become so deformed it looks convex rather than concave.

Motor neuropathy affects the way the muscles work. The muscles actually atrophy. Patients with longstanding diabetes and motor neuropathy may lose as much as half of the muscle volume of their feet. When the muscles of the foot do not work properly, an imbalance occurs and toes are often pulled out of their normal position. These are called hammertoes. When the toes move upward, they also pull with them soft tissue structures like the fat pad on the ball of the foot. This increases pressure on the bottom of the foot, and calluses and ulcers often form. These are deformities that must be addressed.

72

Are there any treatments for peripheral neuropathy?

The best treatment is to keep your blood glucose levels on target. Studies show that near-normal blood glucose levels can also help prevent the nerve damage you already have from getting worse. If you start taking insulin or a sulfonylurea drug to lower your blood glucose, you may notice a short increase in pain until your body becomes accustomed to the lower blood glucose levels.

Medications such as antidepressants, anticonvulsants (seizure medicine), muscle relaxants, local anesthetics (such as a lidocaine patch), and anti-inflammatory drugs, as well as vitamins, evening primrose oil, and capsaicin creams made from hot peppers, have been used to treat neuropathy symptoms. Some doctors have reported success with surgery performed on affected nerves. Physical therapy treatments such as stretching exercises, massage, and electrical nerve stimulation have also been tried. Although studies of these therapies report some improvement in painful symptoms for some patients, there is no single treatment that works for everyone. It may be difficult to get complete relief. Discuss your symptoms with your provider and try the treatment you both think might work. If that treatment doesn't help, let your provider know so you can try another one.

73

How can capsaicin cream help relieve my neuropathy pain?

Capsaicin is a substance found in hot peppers. Capsaicin cream removes a chemical, called substance P, from the nerve ends below your skin and may interrupt your feeling of pain. Apply it lightly several (3 to 4) times a day. Wash your hands carefully after applying capsaicin—you would not want to get hot pepper cream in your eyes, your mouth, or any other sensitive area! When you first use capsaicin, you may have a stinging or burning sensation that should disappear in a few days to a few weeks. Don't give up just because it burns.

Do not use capsaicin if you are sensitive or allergic to hot peppers. Capsaicin cannot be used on damaged or irritated skin, wounds, or rashes. Don't put tight clothing or bandages over the cream. Use it 3 to 4 times a day for 3 to 4 weeks before deciding whether it is working. Since capsaicin comes in different strengths, discuss what strength to use with your health care provider.

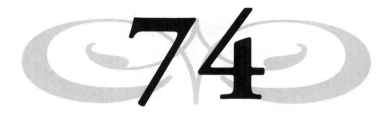

My feet are getting more sensitive, not less. How can this be nerve damage?

When the nerves are in the process of being damaged, many strange signals can be sent up the nerve pathways, including the feeling that your feet are more sensitive than they should be. Some people find it painful for bed sheets to touch their feet. If you experience this sensation, placing a hoop or a box over the end of the bed so that the sheet is kept off your feet might provide you some relief.

Even though your feet may hurt, they can be numb at the same time, and you may not feel when they are being injured. Examine your feet daily and call your foot specialist at the earliest sign of trouble.

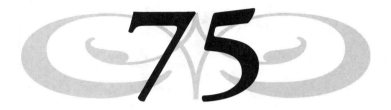

What can I do for the numbness in my feet?

This is a very serious condition. The main thing to do about numbness in your feet is to realize that you have it. Most people go to the doctor because their feet hurt. Yours never will. You must check your feet by touching them with your hands and by looking at them every day! Keeping your blood glucose on target may help prevent the numbness from getting worse. See your podiatrist regularly. Get your shoes fitted properly, if necessary by a pedorthist (certified shoe fitter), and find out whether you need special shoes to protect your feet. Check your shoes before each wearing for foreign objects, nails, or anything that could injure your foot. Be sure your socks are not wrinkled or twisted. You may want to switch to socks without a toe seam, because seams can put too much pressure on your toes.

If you find that the numbness is uncomfortable, discuss treatments for neuropathy with your health care provider. Whenever there is any injury to your feet or a change in shape or a change in the skin, see your foot care specialist right away. Do not wait until an infection develops!

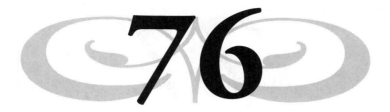

Why does it feel like my feet are burning or tingling—or like something is crawling on them when nothing is there?

Burning, tingling, or crawling sensations on the feet or legs may be a sign that diabetic nerve damage is occurring. The first thing to do is to make sure that there is no obvious cause for this sensation. If you find this sensation uncomfortable, you may want to talk with your health care provider about possible treatments for neuropathy. You may also want to go over your diabetes care plan to see whether it is helping you keep your blood glucose levels where you want them to be.

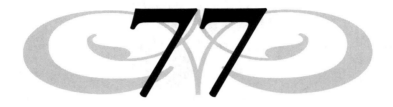

My feet are sweating more. What can I do?

An increase in sweating may be a sign that your blood glucose levels are not on target. Most of the time, diabetic nerve disease decreases foot sweating. Other problems, such as obesity, infectious diseases, hormonal changes associated with menopause, and increased thyroid function, can cause hyperhidrosis (increased sweating). If you have sweaty feet, wear shoes made of leather or fabric that "breathes." Avoid shoes made of plastic or synthetic materials. Try to change your shoes during the day. If that is not possible, rotate between two pairs of shoes, wearing one pair every other day. (Keeping your feet dry helps prevent fungal infections, but you should avoid excessively dry skin that may crack.)

Wear socks that wick the moisture away from your skin (special acrylic blends or CoolMax). Change socks frequently: at least daily and maybe two or three times a day if necessary. If you have to wear nylon stockings, change into socks as soon as you can. Can you wear cotton tights instead?

You may have to try an antiperspirant. Try a regular underarm antiperspirant first. If that doesn't work, you may need a prescription antiperspirant, such as "Drysol." Follow the directions on the package and stop using the product immediately if you experience any skin irritation.

78

Why don't my feet sweat anymore?

A decrease in foot sweating can be a sign that diabetic nerve damage is occurring in the nerves that control sweating. They just don't work normally. This is called autonomic neuropathy. However, foot sweating also tends to decrease as we age, especially if we become less active. Wearing different shoes or socks can affect foot sweating, too. You may have recently started wearing shoes that do not hold in moisture, so your feet are drier.

The problem with a decrease in foot sweating, whatever the cause, is that the foot skin tends to become very dry and prone to cracking. It is a good idea to use a moisturizing cream or lotion on your feet (but not between the toes) if you have dry skin.

79

Why do my feet bother me more at night?

Nobody really knows the answer to this question. It is thought that the symptoms of diabetic nerve damage (pain, burning, tingling, numbness, etc.) are just more noticeable at night because the nerves of the feet and legs are not getting the other signals that they get during the day when you are up and about and walking more. During the day, you also get a broad spectrum of sensory signals from things you see, hear, taste, touch, and smell that keep you busy and distracted from the neuropathy symptoms.

80

Can an unsteady gait be related to diabetic nerve damage?

Yes! When a person has loss of feeling in his or her feet, the positioning system of the body does not get normal responses about where the feet are being placed. This can cause the person to feel unsteady or to trip and stumble. An unsteady gait can be a sign of other problems, too—some of which can be quite serious. If you are having trouble with your balance or walking, talk with your provider about a consultation with a neurologist.

If your trouble is due to nerve damage, it may be time to get a cane. It's better to be safe and use a walking aid than to risk a fall and a broken hip! Your provider or physical therapist can help you get the right length and give you tips on how to walk with a cane. A physical therapist can also teach you balance exercises and how to increase awareness of the position of your feet.

Sometimes diabetes-related muscle weakness can contribute to unsteadiness in walking. Your provider or physical therapist can show you muscle-strengthening exercises. Some people need a lightweight brace or ankle support to stabilize the ankles when muscle weakness is the problem.

81

Two of my toes—the middle toe and the toe next to my baby toe—tingle, burn, and hurt. At first, I had this problem only when I wore tight shoes, but now it is becoming worse, and these toes hurt in any shoes. If I take my shoes off and rub my toes, they feel better. Is this diabetic nerve damage?

Probably not. Compression of a nerve in this area, between the third and fourth toes, causes the nerve to thicken and creates the symptoms you describe. This is called a neuroma (sometimes called Morton's neuroma). People with and without diabetes may get neuromas. Treatment for this problem may include shoe inserts (orthotics), wider shoes, injections of cortisone, injections of alcohol to "kill" the nerve, or surgery either to release pressure on the nerve or to remove the neuroma entirely.

Your question, however, is a perfect example of why an accurate diagnosis from a foot specialist is important. Just because you have diabetes does not mean that diabetes causes every problem you have with your feet (or any other part of your body, for that matter). Treatment for neuromas is generally successful—unless this painful condition is mistakenly treated as diabetic neuropathy.

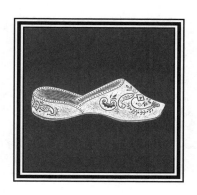

Chapter 9
Complications—
Poor Circulation

82

How do I know when I have poor circulation in my feet and legs?

The hallmark sign of poor circulation is pain or cramping in the calf or the thigh (usually the calf) that occurs when you walk a short distance. This pain is a sign that the muscles are not getting enough oxygen. If you slow or stop and rest for a few minutes, the oxygen supply usually catches up with the demand and then you can walk a little further before the pain reoccurs. The medical term for this condition is "intermittent claudication."

Other signs of poor circulation can be pain at rest, nonhealing ulcers, absent or weak pulses in the feet or legs, a decrease in blood pressure in the feet and legs, or a lack of hair growth on the lower legs. A blue or purplish color, especially when your feet are hanging down, and having cold feet are also signs of circulation problems.

If you think you have poor circulation to the feet, ask your provider to evaluate it. Poor circulation is caused by a blockage in the arteries supplying blood to the feet. The blockage may need to be removed or bypassed with vascular surgery. A simple treatment is to walk every day. This exercise can force the blood vessels to expand and improve the circulation in your feet and legs. Having poor circulation in your feet also puts you at greater risk for heart disease.

83

I have varicose veins. Does that mean I have poor circulation?

Varicose veins are a different type of poor circulation—a poor return of blood to the heart. Your feet are supplied with blood by arteries that carry blood down to them. Veins carry blood from the feet back to the heart. When you stand up, gravity tends to pull blood down toward your feet. Leg veins have valves in them to prevent this from happening. However, if the valves are damaged or too far apart, they do not close properly. This causes varicose veins, which tend to get very full and widen with blood. Varicose veins may look like blue snakes or rivers under the skin. Some of the fluid in the blood leaks out through very small veins (capillaries) and causes swelling. This pooling of blood can cause ulcers on the legs, but these are different from diabetic foot ulcers. Anyone can have varicose veins and leg ulcers.

Wearing support hose and exercising are the two main treatments for varicose veins. Support hose squeeze your legs and prevent blood from pooling in the veins. Exercise also helps keep blood from pooling. When your leg muscles contract, they squeeze nearby veins and help pump blood back to the heart. Surgery is reserved for very severe cases of varicose veins.

84

I have heard that people with diabetes should not have surgery on their feet. Is that true?

Absolutely not. Surgical correction of foot deformities is often your best defense against ulceration, infection, and amputation. A hammertoe, for example, may rub against a neighboring toe or against the inside of the shoe, forming a corn or callus. These hard layers of skin precede most ulcers. The pressure forms an ulcer that, in turn, may become infected and require amputation. If surgery is performed before the ulcer and infection can occur, the toe, foot, or leg may be saved. Any surgery entails some risk, but so does not having a deformity corrected. Nonsurgical care often does not address the true problem and may be only temporary in nature.

Of course, you need good circulation to heal any surgery. Because people with diabetes often develop circulation problems sooner than the general population, your doctor may recommend that you have foot surgery sooner rather than later. Before surgery, your foot surgeon should evaluate your circulation, discuss your diabetes management with you, and explain the postoperative care you will need to follow. If you have any doubts about the suggested surgery, get a second opinion from another qualified foot specialist.

85

My feet are cold. Does this mean I have poor circulation? How can I warm them up?

Many things can cause cold feet. It may be a sign of poor circulation, but it is not a reliable sign. If you think you have poor circulation, have your feet evaluated by your health care provider.

The best thing to do for cold feet is to wear one or two pairs of thick socks or warm house slippers—but check to be sure that your shoes are not too tight. You can try the thin silk socks that are worn under regular socks for added warmth. Getting up and walking around or getting regular exercise helps keep your feet warmer, too.

Do not use heating pads or hot water bottles on your feet. Don't sit too close to a space heater, fireplace, or campfire. If you have any diabetic nerve damage, you cannot feel when your feet are too hot or are getting burned, and you could be badly injured.

In addition to making your feet feel cold, nerve damage can affect blood flow and sweating in the feet. People with these problems are not able to release heat from their feet by dilating blood vessels the way someone without nerve damage would. It's best to wear socks and move around from time to time.

86

One or both of my feet are red, blue, purple, or darker than they used to be. What do these colors mean?

Changes in the color of the skin on your feet can mean many things, from having gangrene to having the dye from your socks rub off. Generally, a color change alone does not tell you enough to know whether it is caused by any specific disease.

Your health care provider will want to evaluate the color change along with other signs and symptoms. She or he will look at your skin, check the pulses in your feet, feel the temperature of your skin, check for infections and broken bones, and evaluate the blood circulation to your feet and legs.

87

What is peripheral vascular disease?

Peripheral vascular disease (PVD) is commonly called "poor circulation" and refers to blockage in the blood supply to the feet. A buildup of plaque inside the arteries that carry blood to the feet causes them to thicken and harden. People without diabetes get this thickening and hardening of the arteries, too, but unfortunately these problems can happen sooner and can be more severe in people with diabetes. PVD is 20 times more common in people with diabetes than in the general population. Other things that put you at risk of developing PVD are smoking, poor nutrition, lack of exercise, high blood fat levels (including cholesterol), and high blood glucose levels. Women are just as much at risk, and young as well as older people can develop it.

You can help to avoid or limit PVD by stopping smoking and keeping your blood fats and blood glucose levels as close to normal as possible. See a registered dietitian (RD) for help with your meal plan and add more physical activity to your lifestyle.

88

What kind of tests do I need for PVD?

Your health care provider will ask questions about your symptoms. He or she will examine your feet and legs and feel for pulses, located in the groin, behind the knee, at the ankle, and on top of the foot. You may need to have the blood pressure in your ankles, arms, legs, and toes checked. (The arteries in toes don't get stiff, so measuring blood pressure there may be more accurate.) A Doppler machine may be used; this test is painless. You may need a test to measure how much oxygen gets to the skin of your feet. If you have an ulcer that won't heal or areas of your foot that break down despite wearing properly fitted shoes, you may need tests such as special X-rays and scans. These tests give pictures of the blood flow from your thigh to your toes. For arteriogram X-rays, you get an intravenous injection of a special solution so that the blood vessels show up clearly on the X-ray. This solution is called "dye," although it really does not change the color of anything. People with poor circulation should consult with a vascular surgeon, a doctor who specializes in this type of problem. If you have questions, ask your provider and the people performing the tests to explain things to you.

89

How often should I have my foot circulation checked?

Your physician and your podiatrist should check your foot and ankle pulses at every visit. If the pulses are decreased or absent, further testing may be needed.

People with diabetes who are over the age of 50 should have a baseline Doppler exam (also called an ankle/arm index) to compare the blood pressure in their feet and arms. If the test is normal—that is, if your ankle pressure is equal to or above your arm pressure—the test should be repeated every five years. If the initial test is abnormal, you may need additional tests, or you may be referred to a vascular surgeon (circulation specialist) for treatment.

90

What does smoking have to do with my feet?

Smoking is clearly connected to developing vascular (heart and blood vessel) disease. When you smoke, the combustion products of tobacco are absorbed into the bloodstream. These chemicals stimulate the release of other chemicals, which injure the blood vessels and encourage thickening and hardening of the arteries. Smoking also causes your blood vessels to constrict or clamp down, limiting the amount of blood that can circulate. Smoking even as few as two cigarettes a day can constrict the blood vessels all day long.

Smoking and diabetes are a deadly combination for the vascular system. If you have diabetes and smoke you are greatly increasing the risk of amputation!

Fortunately, there are many new medications and good programs to help people quit smoking. If you smoke and you're ready to quit, ask your health care provider to refer you to one of these programs to help you do it.

91

Are there any treatments for PVD?

Preventing vascular disease is much easier than treating it. That is why your health care provider will stress that you quit smoking, keep your blood pressure and blood glucose on target, control your cholesterol and triglycerides, lose weight, and stay active. Your doctor can prescribe some medications to treat PVD. Taking an aspirin a day can help prevent heart attacks and strokes, so some people think that it might help prevent PVD, too. Aspirin is not recommended for everyone and can interact with other medications you may be taking, so ask your provider before you start taking aspirin daily.

If you have intermittent claudication (pain in your calves with walking), you might be asked to walk more. Usually you are encouraged to walk to the point of pain, pause, and then walk a little more. Ask your provider to give you instructions. Walking may help stimulate new vessels to grow and this will improve circulation.

92

Will I need surgery for PVD?

If the tests for PVD show that you have blockage in the larger arteries to your feet or legs, surgeons may try to correct it. One surgery cleans out the artery that is blocked. Another method, called angioplasty, involves passing a deflated balloon on a tube to the point where the blockage occurs. Then the balloon is carefully inflated to open the narrowed artery, and sometimes a stent (a tiny metal device shaped like a spring) is inserted in the artery to keep it open. This surgery is most successful with a small blockage in a healthy artery. A third surgical method is to bypass the blocked area by using a blood vessel from another part of the body (or an artificial blood vessel). While complicated, this surgery can help save a foot. People with diabetes often have many blockages in the arteries of the lower legs and feet, making it difficult to restore circulation. The relatively new ability to do bypass surgery down to the small arteries of the foot has saved many legs. Not all vascular surgeons do this surgery, so check to be sure that yours can. Your providers will carefully evaluate your condition before recommending surgery.

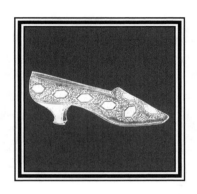

Chapter 10
Other Foot Problems

93

I have arthritis in my foot. How is it going to react with diabetes?

Arthritis is defined as inflammation of a joint usually characterized by swelling, pain, and restriction of motion. There are different kinds of arthritis and different treatments for each kind. It is best to let your health care provider diagnose and treat any problems you are having with your joints. Don't assume that any pain, swelling, or stiffness in your foot is "just arthritis." There are many over-the-counter medications for treating arthritis, but consult your health care provider if you take these regularly.

Since both arthritis and diabetes tend to affect people as they age, it is common to have both conditions. Arthritis can make it difficult for people with diabetes to stay as active as they need to be. However, because exercising and staying active are treatments for both arthritis and diabetes, you get a double dose of benefits whenever you exercise.

There are many new medications for arthritis. The current thinking is that arthritis should be treated more aggressively than it was in years past. Researchers think that starting treatment early could prevent much of the pain and disability associated with arthritis.

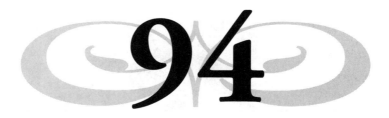

I have gout in my foot. How is it going to react with diabetes?

Gout is a special type of arthritis caused by an excess of uric acid in the blood. Uric acid crystals tend to settle in joints; the big toe or bunion joint is the most common site. These crystals can cause the big toe joint to become extremely painful, red, warm, and swollen. If you have the symptoms of gout, your health care provider may withdraw some joint fluid and examine it under a microscope to look for these crystals. Medications and a special diet to lower the uric acid levels in the body are the main treatments for gout.

Sometimes it is difficult to tell the difference between gout and an infection caused by bacteria. If you think you might have gout, it is important to see your health care provider.

Repeated episodes of gout tend to damage the big toe joint and may make it stiff. This can cause a high-pressure spot on your foot that is more prone to developing a callus and an ulcer. Be sure to check your feet daily for any signs of redness or ulceration. If the joint does become stiff, you may need surgery to help loosen it or to replace it with an artificial joint.

95

What is Charcot's joint and how do I recognize it?

Charcot's joint or Charcot foot is the term used to describe a severe deformity in a weight-bearing joint. A French physician named J. M. Charcot first described it in the 1860s. Charcot foot refers to the breakdown of the arch and normal foot structure in a person with nerve damage. Because Charcot's joint usually happens to people who have nerve damage, there is not much pain, even though they may have broken bones. There may be redness, swelling, and increased warmth of the foot. Your shoes won't fit. That's when people usually go to see their provider. Stay off that foot. The breakdown may occur fairly quickly. Sometimes it is difficult to tell the difference between Charcot's joint and infection. Your foot specialist may order special tests, such as MRIs or bone scans, to make a definitive diagnosis.

Treatments for Charcot's joint are to immobilize the foot in a cast or special boot and rest the foot so it can heal. Sometimes surgery is done to realign the joints of the foot. If you continue to walk on a foot with Charcot's joint, you will make it much worse. If you can't get your regular shoes on, or if you have any changes in foot shape along with redness, swelling, or warmth, contact your health care provider immediately.

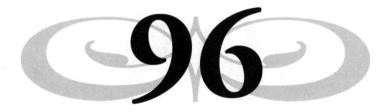

Having a foot deformity is listed as a major risk factor for amputation. What exactly is a foot deformity?

A foot deformity is any change in the normal shape of the foot. For people with diabetes, a deformity may be complicated by the additional risk factors of poor sensation and poor circulation. It is the combination of these factors that can make foot deformities dangerous.

Common deformities include bunions (enlargements of the bone just behind the big toe), hammertoes, claw toes or mallet toes (a bending of the toe bones upward), curving of the toes toward each other, tailor's bunions (enlargements of the bone just behind the little toe), enlargements or bumps of bone behind the heels or on the top or bottom of the foot, and Charcot deformities, which may look like a collapsing of the foot at the arch.

Discuss the options for treatment of any deformity with your foot specialist. If you have adequate circulation, your best bet may be surgery to fix the deformity. Alternatives to surgery include special pads or cushions that may be off-the-shelf or custom-made, shoes with extra depth and specially fabricated innersoles, or even custom-made shoes.

97

What is osteomyelitis, and how do I recognize it?

Osteomyelitis is the medical name for an infection in the bone. If you have a foot ulcer that is not healing well, your health care provider will want to examine your foot with an X-ray, an MRI, or a bone scan to determine whether the nearby bones have been affected. This is important because the treatments for bone infection and for soft tissue infection are different. It is also extremely difficult to heal foot ulcers over infected bone. Surgery is sometimes required to remove the infected bone.

If you notice an ulcer during your daily foot exams, be sure to call your podiatrist at once. Early treatment may prevent the onset of osteomyelitis. Since osteomyelitis often occurs in areas with ulcers, prevention of ulcers is extremely important.

98

I may have osteomyelitis in my foot. My doctor is running many expensive tests. Are they necessary?

Unfortunately, an infection of a bone (osteomyelitis) is a serious medical problem. If an infection is present, it must be treated aggressively with surgery, antibiotics, or both. Getting an accurate diagnosis is important, but diabetes can complicate the diagnostic process.

Sometimes, people with diabetes have a problem that looks like a bone infection but really isn't. Diabetes and diabetic neuropathy affect the way bones look on X-rays, and they can cause redness, swelling, and warmth similar to those that occur with bone infections. This similarity can make diagnosis difficult.

Your doctor may order a number of tests to help with the diagnosis. A bone biopsy is the best test, but it requires surgical removal of a small piece of bone. The bone is examined for signs of infection, and then it is cultured to determine which antibiotic will work best. Other, nonsurgical tests that may be used include bone scans, bone scans with labeled white blood cells, and MRIs. These are all expensive tests, but they are often necessary to differentiate osteomyelitis from other problems. Your podiatrist, along with specialists in infectious disease, orthopedics, and radiology, can and should answer all your questions about each test ordered.

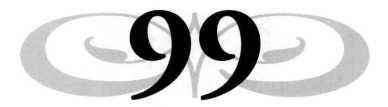

What is gangrene? What causes it?

Gangrene is a term that refers to death of the skin and the underlying tissues. It is usually caused by poor blood flow to an injured area and may be followed by infection. The area of gangrene usually becomes dark brown or black. Once the tissue is dead, it will not grow back.

Sometimes when a toe becomes gangrenous, it may be left to just dry up and fall off. Other times the gangrene may be spreading and may need to be removed by surgery. You may need bypass surgery to improve circulation, which will help stop the gangrene from spreading, preserve as much of the toe or foot as possible, and prevent further problems. As gangrene progresses, it may lead to the loss of a toe, foot, leg, or life. To prevent such disasters, all people with diabetes need an appropriate foot care plan.

100

I had to have a toe amputation. Am I doomed?

No, you are not doomed! However, once you have an amputation, you are at much higher risk for having another one. That is why you need to do everything you can to prevent diabetic foot problems. Check your feet daily, have your health care provider check your feet at every visit, see your podiatrist regularly, and try to keep your blood fats and blood glucose levels as close to normal as possible. An amputation can "create" a foot deformity and put unusual pressure on the bones in your foot. You'll need orthotics, padding, or special shoes to be sure that you don't get another ulcer on your foot. You might need physical therapy to learn how to walk smoothly. You may benefit from counseling or from joining a support group of other people who have had amputations. You are likely to feel some pretty strong emotions after an experience like this.

Many people who have had a toe, foot, or leg amputation lead full and active lives. Medical science has made excellent breakthroughs in artificial limbs and rehabilitation for people with amputations. You may want to contact the Amputee Coalition of America (www.amputee-coalition.org), which helps people who have amputations through education and support.

101

What can a person who has had one leg amputated do to prevent amputation of the remaining leg?

Statistically, there is a 28% to 51% chance that a person with diabetes who has had a lower extremity amputation will need a second amputation within 5 years. Obviously, the remaining limb is extremely valuable, and you must protect it as if it were made of gold.

Any amputation puts additional stress on the remaining lower extremity structures. If you have peripheral vascular disease (poor circulation), you may need to correct that problem in your remaining limb. Ask your doctor if you should see a vascular surgeon.

See your podiatrist frequently, and follow any directions carefully. Never walk without protective footgear. You may now need special therapeutic shoes and innersoles. Any foot deformities such as hammertoes or bunions need special attention, now more than ever. Examine your foot at least once a day. If you note any problems or changes, such as ingrown nails, red spots, or any wounds, call your foot specialist at once.

Resources

American Diabetes Association
1701 North Beauregard Street
Alexandria, VA 22311
(800) DIABETES
(703) 549-1500
Website: www.diabetes.org
Bookstore: www.store.diabetes.org

American Academy of Orthopaedic Surgeons
6300 North River Road
Rosemont, IL 60018-4262
(800) 346-AAOS
(847) 823-7186
Website: www.aaos.org

American Association of Diabetes Educators
100 West Monroe, Suite 400
Chicago, IL 60603
(800) 338-3633
Website: www.aadenet.org
E-mail: aade@aadenet.org

American Board of Podiatric Surgery
445 Fillmore Street
San Francisco, CA 94117-3404
(415) 553-7800
Website: www.abps.org
E-mail: info@abps.org

American College of Foot and Ankle Surgeons
8725 West Higgins Road, Suite 555
Chicago, IL 60631
(800) 421-2237
(773) 693-9300
Website: www.acfas.org
E-mail: info@acfas.org

American Orthopaedic Foot and Ankle Society
2517 Eastlake Avenue East, Suite 200
Seattle, WA 98102
(206) 223-1120
(800) 235-4855
Website: www.aofas.org
E-mail: aofas@aofas.org

American Podiatric Medical Association
9312 Old Georgetown Road
Bethesda, MD 20814-1698
(301) 571-9200
(800) FOOTCARE
Website: www.apma.org

Amputee Coalition of America
900 East Hill Avenue, Suite 285
Knoxville, TN 37915-2568
(888) 267-5669
Website: www.amputee-coalition.org

Diabetes Exercise and Sports Association (DESA)
8001 Montcastle Drive
Nashville, TN 37221
(800) 898-4322
Website: www.diabetes-exercise.org
E-mail: desa@diabetes-exercise.org

Lower Extremity Amputation Prevention Program (LEAP)
National Hansen's Disease Programs (NHDP)
1770 Physicians Park Drive
Baton Rouge, LA 70816
(800) 642-2477
Website: bphc.hrsa.gov/leap

National Chronic Pain Outreach Association
P.O. Box 274
Millboro, VA 24460
(540) 862-9437
Website: www.chronicpain.org

National Odd Shoe Exchange
P.O. Box 1120
Chandler, AZ 85244-1120
Website: www.oddshoe.org

Neuropathy Association
60 East 42nd Street, Suite 942
New York, NY 10165
(800) 247-6968
(212) 692-0662
Website: www.neuropathy.org
E-mail: info@neuropathy.org

One Shoe Crew
E-mail: Sally_tvarez@hotmail.com

Pedorthic Footwear Association
7150 Columbia Gateway Drive, Suite G
Columbia, MD 21046-1151
(800) 673-8447
(410) 381-7278
Website: www.pedorthics.org

President's Council on Physical Fitness and Sports
200 Independence Avenue, SW
Room 738-H
Washington, DC 20201-0004
(202) 690-9000
Website: www.fitness.gov

State-Based Diabetes Prevention and Control Programs
Centers for Disease Control
CDC Division of Diabetes Translation
P.O. Box 8728
Silver Spring, MD 20910
(877) 232-3422
Website: www.cdc.gov/diabetes/states/
E-mail: diabetes@cdc.gov

Take Care of Your Feet for a Lifetime (brochure)
National Diabetes Education Program
National Institutes of Health
Website: www.ndep.nih.gov/diabetes/pubs/Feet_broch_Eng.pdf

Index

corns *(continued)*
   between toes, 64
   custom shoes. *See* shoes

D
diabetes care team, 11
diabetes complications, 3, 7
   exercise and, 72
   eye disease, 7
   kidney disease, 7
   nerve damage, 3, 4
   poor circulation, 3, 4, 108
Diabetes Control and
   Complications Trial (DCCT),
   10
diabetic neuropathy. *See* nerve
   damage
diet. *See* meal plan
diuretics, 31
Doppler exam, 110

E
endocrinologist, 11
exercise, 17, 71, 72, 117
   aging and, 17
   diabetes complications and, 72
   nerve damage and, 71, 72
   peripheral vascular disease
      and, 108
   shoes for, 71, 73
   ulcers and, 71
eye problems, 7, 15

F
flexibility, lack of, 16
foot care, 7, 8, 16, 19, 23
   eye problems and, 15
foot care team, 11
foot deformities, 45, 77, 90, 120
   amputation and, 120
   custom shoes for, 50
   surgery for, 105
foot examinations, 13, 14, 19, 110
   frequency of, 13
   poor circulation and, 110
foot infections. *See* infections
foot odor, 29
foot problems
   diabetes complications and, 77
   prevention, 8
   risk factors, 7, 77
foot specialist. *See* podiatrist
foot swelling. *See* swelling
foot ulcer. *See* ulcers
footwear. *See* shoes
fungus, 5, 26. *See also* athlete's
   foot fungus

G
gangrene, 107, 123
gout, 118

H
hammertoes, 8, 77, 90, 105, 120
high blood pressure, 30

I

infections, 4, 5, 82, 84,105

injury. *See* wounds

insoles, 52

intermittent claudication, 103, 112. *See also* circulation, peripheral vascular disease

K

kidney disease, 7
swelling and, 30

M

meal plan, 18, 108

Medicare, 51, 83

moisturizers, 23, 24, 25

monofilament test, 13, 79, 89

Morton's neuroma, 100

motor neuropathy, 87, 90

N

nail clippers, 35, 37

nails. *See* toenails

National Odd Shoe Exchange, 46

nephropathy (kidney disease), 7, 30

nerve damage, 3, 4, 6, 7, 9, 77, 87, 88, 89. *See also* peripheral neuropathy
blisters and, 59
blood glucose levels and, 6, 88
calluses and, 87

cold feet and, 106

custom shoes and, 50

dry skin and, 24, 87

exercise and, 71, 72

foot pain and, 91, 92, 93

incidence of, 89

monofilament test for, 13, 79, 89

numbness and, 94

tuning fork test for, 13, 89

ulcers and, 87

uncomfortable sensations in feet and, 95

neurologist, 11

neuroma, 100

neuropathy. *See* peripheral neuropathy, autonomic neuropathy, nerve damage

numbness, 94

O

obesity, 9

occupational therapist, 11

odor. *See* foot odor

One Shoe Crew, 46

orthopedic surgeon, 12

orthotics, 47, 52, 53

osteomyelitis, 121, 122

P

pain, 4, 91
absence of, 60

About the American Diabetes Association

The American Diabetes Association is the nation's leading voluntary health organization supporting diabetes research, information, and advocacy. Its mission is to prevent and cure diabetes and to improve the lives of all people affected by diabetes. The American Diabetes Association is the leading publisher of comprehensive diabetes information. Its huge library of practical and authoritative books for people with diabetes covers every aspect of self-care—cooking and nutrition, fitness, weight control, medications, complications, emotional issues, and general self-care.

To order American Diabetes Association books: Call 1-800-232-6733 or log on to http://store.diabetes.org

To join the American Diabetes Association: Call 1-800-806-7801 or log on to www.diabetes.org/membership

For more information about diabetes or ADA programs and services: Call 1-800-342-2383. E-mail: AskADA@diabetes.org or log on to www.diabetes.org

To locate an ADA/NCQA Recognized Provider of quality diabetes care in your area: www.ncqa.org/dprp

To find an ADA Recognized Education Program in your area: Call 1-800-342-2383. www.diabetes.org/for-health-professionals-and-scientists/recognition/edrecognition.jsp

To join the fight to increase funding for diabetes research, end discrimination, and improve insurance coverage: Call 1-800-342-2383. www.diabetes.org/advocacy-and-legalresources/advocacy.jsp

To find out how you can get involved with the programs in your community: Call 1-800-342-2383. See below for program Web addresses.

American Diabetes Month: educational activities aimed at those diagnosed with diabetes—month of November. www.diabetes.org/communityprograms-and-localevents/americandiabetesmonth.jsp

American Diabetes Alert: annual public awareness campaign to find the undiagnosed—held the fourth Tuesday in March. www.diabetes.org/communityprograms-and-localevents/americandiabetesalert.jsp

The Diabetes Assistance & Resources Program (DAR): diabetes awareness program targeted to the Latino community. www.diabetes.org/communityprograms-and-localevents/latinos.jsp

African American Program: diabetes awareness program targeted to the African American community. www.diabetes.org/communityprograms-and-localevents/africanamericans.jsp

Awakening the Spirit: Pathways to Diabetes Prevention & Control: diabetes awareness program targeted to the Native American community. www.diabetes.org/communityprograms-and-localevents/nativeamericans.jsp

To find out about an important research project regarding type 2 diabetes: www.diabetes.org/diabetes-research/research-home.jsp

To obtain information on making a planned gift or charitable bequest: Call 1-888-700-7029. www.wpg.cc/stl/CDA/homepage/1,1006,509,00.html

To make a donation or memorial contribution: Call 1-800-342-2383. www.diabetes.org/support-the-cause/make-a-donation.jsp

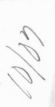